Contents

Normal Infant and Examination (1)

Mongolian blue spot

Incidence
Almost universal in non-Caucasian neonates. Particularly obvious in Asian infants. Occasionally occurs in Caucasian infants with dark hair.

Clinical features
Slate grey or bluish pigmentation, usually in the lumbo-sacral region (Figs 1 & 2) but may occur anywhere on the trunk or limbs (Fig. 3).

Significance
None, except may be mistaken for bruising by the inexperienced.

Course and prognosis
Gradually become less obvious as the infant grows older.

Erythema toxicum

Synonyms
Toxic erythema, urticaria of the newborn, eosinophil rash.

Incidence
Extremely common; majority of newborn infants are affected in the first week of life. Not seen in preterm infants.

Aetiology
Unknown.

Pathology
Vesicles are full of eosinophils.

Clinical features
Widespread, fluctuating erythematous maculo-papular rash (Fig. 4) usually beginning after birth at any time in the first week. Individual lesions consist of a white central papule surrounded by an erythematous flare.

Significance
None, except may occasionally be mistaken for septic spots.

Course
Disappears spontaneously.

Treatment
None required.

NEONATOLOGY

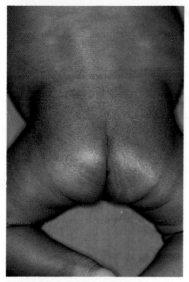

Fig. 1 Typical Mongolian blue spot in lumbo-sacral region.

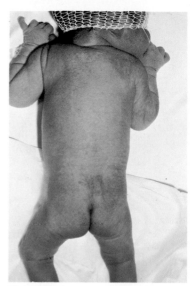

Fig. 2 More extensive Monogolian blue spot.

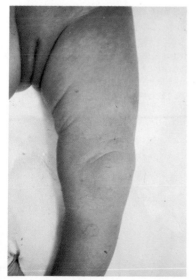

Fig. 3 Mongolian blue spot around the knee.

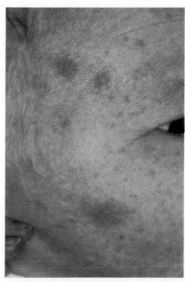

Fig. 4 Erythema toxicum on the face.

Normal Infant and Examination (2)

Vernix caseosum

Incidence

Common.

Clinical features

Slimy, ointment-like white substance on the skin of some infants at birth. Usually found around the face (Fig. 5), ears and in the folds of the neck or groin (Fig. 6), but is occasionally liberally caked all over the body. Vernix is sometimes stained by meconium if there was fetal distress some time before birth.

Significance

None.
Vernix is more common towards the end of gestation, but tends to disappear after term.

Course

Dries and flakes off within a few hours after birth.

Treatment

None required.

Vascular phenomena

Incidence

Very common.

Aetiology

Innocent manifestation of vasomotor instability or immaturity.

Clinical features

Peripheral cyanosis is very common in the first 48 h after birth (Fig. 7). It occurs in the extremities and around the mouth. There is no central cyanosis. Harlequin colour change is a very rare, but dramatic colour change with vivid midline demarcation of colour. The infant is red on one side of the trunk and pale on the other side.

Treatment

None required.

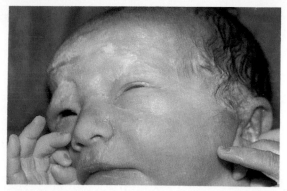

Fig. 5 Vernix caseosum on face.

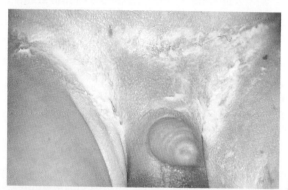

Fig. 6 Vernix caseosum in the groins.

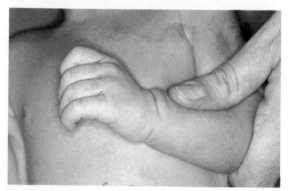

Fig. 7 Peripheral cyanosis of the hand in a normal full-term baby.

Normal Infant and Examination (3)

Milia and epithelial pearls

Synonyms	Milia, milk spots, epithelial pearls.
Incidence	Very common; seen in 40–50% of newborn infants.
Pathology	Milia are hypertrophic sebaceous glands. Epithelial pearls are epidermal cysts.
Clinical features	Milia are fine white spots seen on the nose (Fig. 8) and cheeks. Epithelial pearls occur as a cluster of several white spots in the mouth at the junction of the soft and hard palate in the midline (Fig. 9). Less commonly, they occur on the alveolar margin or on the prepuce.
Significance	None, but occasionally mistaken for infection.
Course and prognosis	Disappear spontaneously.

Ranula

Incidence	Uncommon.
Clinical features	Superficial mucous retention cyst in the anterior part of the floor of the mouth, under the tongue (Fig. 10). Deeper cysts may occur in relation to the submandibular or sublingual ducts.
Management	Often disappear spontaneously. Large cysts may occasionally interfere with feeding and surgery may then be indicated (marsupialisation).

Natal teeth

Incidence	Uncommon, but there is often a family history of similar teeth.
Clinical features	Commonly occur in the central lower incisor region (Fig. 11) and usually only loosely attached.
Management	Best removed early in order to prevent aspiration or ulceration of the tongue. Extraction will not deplete the permanent dentition.

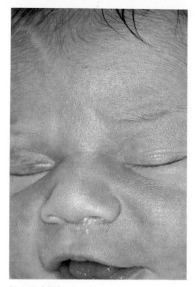

Fig. 8 Milia on nose.

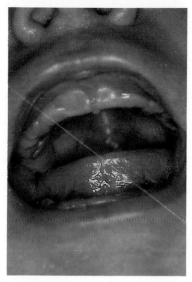

Fig. 9 Epithelial pearls in the midline of the palate.

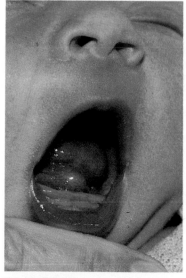

Fig. 10 Ranula.

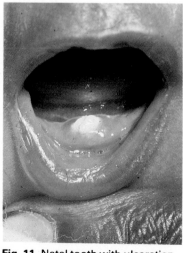

Fig. 11 Natal tooth with ulceration underneath the tongue.

Normal Infant and Examination (4)

Simple naevus

Synonym	Stork bite naevus.
Incidence	Very common. Seen in 30–50% of infants.
Pathology	Capillary haemangioma.
Clinical features	Bright pink macular capillary haemangiomata seen on the eyelids, bridge of the nose, upper lip (Fig. 12) and nape of the neck (Fig. 13). On the forehead, there is sometimes a V-shaped lesion said in folklore to be the mark of the stork's beak. Simple naevi do not blanch on pressure.
Significance	None.
Course and prognosis	All simple naevi on the face disappear spontaneously in the first year. Those on the nape of the neck are usually permanent, but never require treatment.

Sucking pad

Synonym	Sucking callous.
Incidence	Common.
Clinical features	Dry thickened epithelium of the mucous membranes of the lips (Fig. 14) in the first few weeks of life. Often form a discrete pad or callous.
Aetiology	Unknown, but not related to pressure or trauma as they can occur in the absence of sucking and are often present at birth.
Significance	None.
Management	None required. They disappear spontaneously.

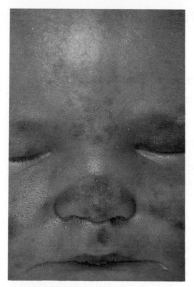

Fig. 12 Simple naevus on eyelids, nose and upper lip.

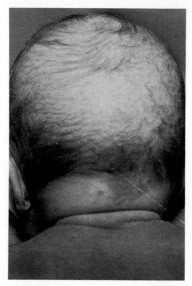

Fig. 13 Simple naevus on nape of the neck.

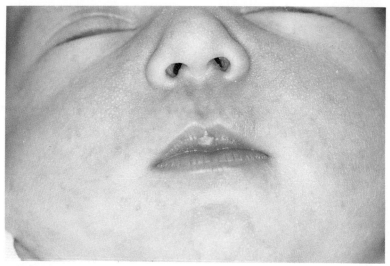

Fig. 14 Sucking pad on lip.

Normal Infant and Examination (5)

Hormonal manifestations— gynaecomastia and vaginal bleeding

Incidence

Very common.
The majority of newborn infants have palpable breast nodules and 30–40% have obvious gynaecomastia.
Both sexes may have gynaecomastia.

Aetiology

Probably due to placental transfer of maternal oestrogen, progesterone and prolactin.

Clinical features

Breast enlargement, often with lactation (witch's milk) is present during the first weeks of life. In hormonal gynaecomastia, there is no evidence of inflammation (Fig. 15). Erythema only occurs when the breast has become infected (mastitis). Vaginal bleeding, or a discharge of mucus (Fig. 16), occurs in some infants a few days after birth.

Course

Gradual involution of the breast tissue occurs, but may take some months to disappear.

Management

No treatment is required for hormonal gynaecomastia and vaginal bleeding. Reassurance and explanation of the physiological nature of these events should be given to the parents. Do not squeeze the breasts to express milk. Antibiotics are only necessary if the breast becomes infected.

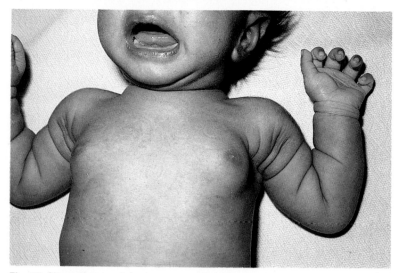

Fig. 15 Normal neonatal gynaecomastia.

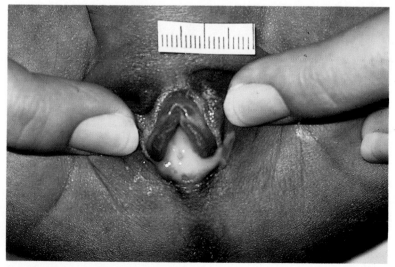

Fig. 16 Normal mucoid vaginal discharge.

Normal Infant and Examination (6)

Sacral pits and dimples

Incidence	Common.
Clinical features	Pits or dimples are often present over the sacrum (Fig. 17) and a prominent coccyx can often be palpated in the base.
Significance	They are usually trivial and blind-ending. Fistulae can usually be excluded by careful inspection; otherwise radiological investigation may be necessary.
Associations	Other midline abnormalities such as haemangiomata, hairy naevi or lipomas may occur. They are usually situated higher on the back and may be associated with tethering of the cauda equina (diastatomyelia).
Management	None required, if fistula has been excluded.

Vulval tag

Incidence	Common.
Clinical features	A tag of mucous membrane is often present in the posterior vulval region of newborn female infants (Fig. 18). It is often long and pedunculated.
Significance	None.
Course and prognosis	Shrivels up and disappears spontaneously within a few days of birth
Treatment	None required.

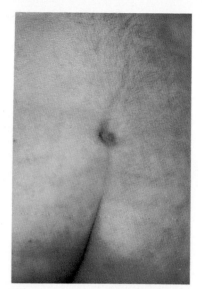

Fig. 17 A dimple over sacrum.

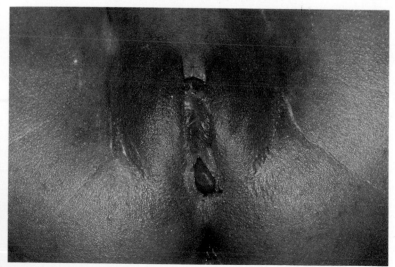

Fig. 18 Posterior vulval tag.

Normal Infant and Examination (7)

Umbilical cord

Clinical features

The umbilical cord usually has a fleshy translucent appearance in the first days after birth. It is sometimes stained yellow or greenish-yellow with bilirubin in rhesus haemolytic disease or meconium if there has been fetal distress. The normal umbilical cord contains two arteries and one vein (Fig. 19). A single umbilical artery may be associated with other congenital abnormalities.

Course

The cord gradually separates within 7–10 days after birth, either by dry gangrene (Fig. 20) or with a residual moist base (Fig. 21). Frank discharge or cellulitis with a red flare around the umbilicus indicate infection and require treatment with systemic antibiotics after culture.
Persistent sero-sanguinous discharge or a fleshy protuberance from the base may indicate the development of an umbilical granuloma. The presence of a vitello-intestinal remnant or persistent urachus should be excluded. A granuloma can be readily treated with the local application of silver nitrate or rarely by surgical excision.

Management

Gentle cleaning with a spirit swab is all that is required for the normal moist umbilical cord until spontaneous separation occurs. The application of topical antibiotics may actually delay separation. Prolonged adherence of the umbilical cord beyond 3 weeks of age has been associated with a rare disorder of granulocyte function.

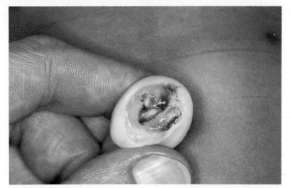

Fig. 19 Cut surface of umbilical cord showing two arteries and one vein.

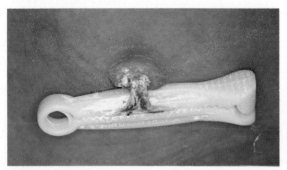

Fig. 20 Dry cord.

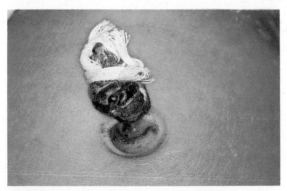

Fig. 21 Separating cord with a moist base.

Normal Infant and Examination (8)

Stools

Meconium

Sticky, tarry, greenish-black stool (Fig. 22) passed by the newborn infant within the first 48 h after birth. Failure to pass meconium within 48 h of birth may indicate intestinal obstruction. Meconium is odourless and consists of mucus, epithelial debris and bile from the gastro-intestinal tract before feeding. Meconium may be passed by the fetus before birth if there is fetal distress. Inhalation of meconium results in pneumonitis with severe respiratory distress, and vigorous suction and resuscitation are indicated immediately after delivery before the first spontaneous breath.

Changing stool

With the onset of feeding, the stools gradually change in colour and consistency (Fig. 23). They become softer, greenish in colour and mixed with mucus for a few days.

Breast fed baby's stools

Mustard yellow or greenish-yellow in colour and only a faint sweet odour. Breast fed stools are usually soft and semi-formed (Fig. 24) but are sometimes liquid. Frequency varies, but they are often passed after or during each feed.

Bottle fed baby's stools

Usually firmer, browner and passed less frequently than those of a breast fed infant. The appearance and odour vary considerably, but in general they are more like a normal adult stool.

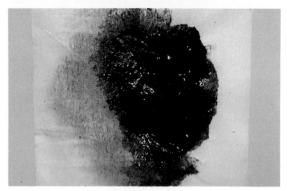

Fig. 22 Meconium.

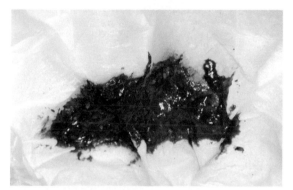

Fig. 23 Changing stool.

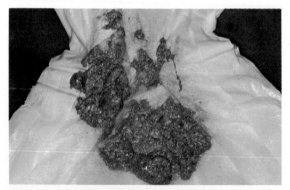

Fig. 24 Breast fed baby's stool.

Normal Infant and Examination (9)

Jaundice

Incidence

Very common; 50% of full-term infants and 80% of preterm infants are visibly jaundiced by 3–5 days of age.

1. *Physiological jaundice* appears after 48 h of birth and usually settles within 7–10 days. It is mainly unconjugated bilirubin due to increased red cell destruction and immaturity of hepatic enzymes.
2. *Early jaundice* occurring within 24–48 h of birth is usually due to abnormal haemolysis, infection or bruising from birth trauma.
3. *Prolonged jaundice* lasting beyond 14 days is sometimes seen in normal preterm or breast fed infants but other conditions should be excluded; especially hypothyroidism, galactosaemia, liver disease, red cell enzyme defects and biliary atresia.

Clinical features

Yellow staining of the skin (Fig. 25) and conjunctivae. Hepatosplenomegaly indicates the presence of abnormal haemolysis, infection or a metabolic disorder, and is not found in physiological jaundice.

Significance

Very severe unconjugated hyperbilirubinaemia may cause permanent brain damage (kernicterus).

Management

Observe jaundice clinically and monitor plasma bilirubin level. Investigation may be required if jaundice appears earlier than 48 h, is prolonged beyond 14 days or is unusually high at any stage. Dehydration and drugs such as sulphonamides which compete with bilirubin for albumin-binding should be avoided. There is no evidence that extra fluids are needed or hasten the resolution of jaundice in normal infants. Phototherapy (Fig. 26) or exchange transfusion may be required in some infants with high levels of plasma bilirubin. Some jaundiced babies develop a curious bronze colour under phototherapy (Fig. 27).

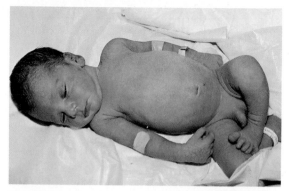

Fig. 25 Jaundice due to unconjugated bilirubinaemia.

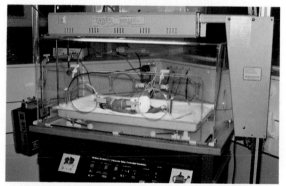

Fig. 26 Phototherapy.

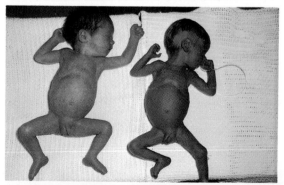

Fig. 27 Bronze baby syndrome with a normal baby.

Neonatal reflexes

Occurrence

The normal newborn infant has a large number of primitive neurological reflexes which disappear spontaneously during early infancy. The presence or absence may be useful in the assessment of gestational age and neurological function. Delayed disappearance of certain primitive reflexes may be an early sign of cerebral palsy.

Clinical features

Moro or startle reflex
The infant is held supine, with trunk and head being supported from below. When the head and shoulders are suddenly allowed to fall back, a startle response with rapid abduction and extension of the upper limbs followed by slower adduction and flexion is elicited. The Moro reflex is often accompanied by a cry and may be demonstrated unintentionally when briskly placing an infant in the supine position (Fig. 28). Babies do not seem to like the reflex, so it should not be elicited as a routine procedure. The commonest cause of an asymmetric Moro response is a fracture of the humerus or clavicle, or a brachial plexus palsy.

Grasp reflexes
Flexion of the digits is a positive response to a finger being placed on the palmar surface of the base of the fingers (Fig. 29) or the plantar surface of the toes.

Sucking and rooting reflexes
Stroking the face around the mouth or cheek causes a reflex sucking (Fig. 30) and searching response.

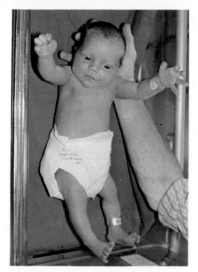

Fig. 28 Moro or startle reflex.

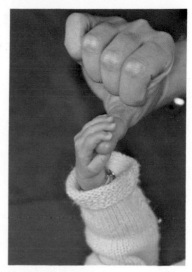

Fig. 29 Grasp reflex.

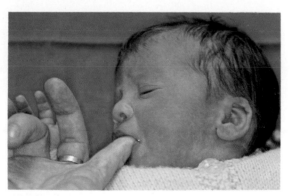

Fig. 30 Sucking response.

Neonatal reflexes (contd)

**Clinical
features
(contd)**

Glabellar tap
A blink of the eyelids is produced in response to tapping the base of the nose.

Traction reflex
Pulling the infant up from the supine position by the wrists results in flexion of the arms and neck.

Placing reflex
If the foot is brought up gently under the edge of a surface, the leg is flexed and the baby places the foot on to the surface.

Walking reflex
When the sole of the foot is brought into contact with a surface, there is an automatic walking movement (Fig. 31).

Galant reflex
If the posterior loin is stroked, the baby swings the buttock towards that side.

Asymmetric tonic neck reflex
If the head is turned laterally, there is extension of the arm and leg on the same side and flexion of the opposite arm and leg (Fig. 32).

Significance

Only very general conclusions can be drawn from examination of an infant for primitive reflexes. None of the reflexes is associated with a particular anatomical or pathological lesion. Their presence or absence must be considered in association with the history, gestational age and other aspects of the neurological examination.

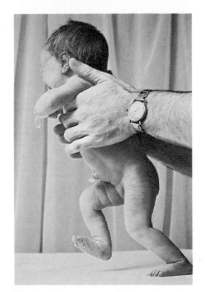

Fig. 31 Automatic walking.

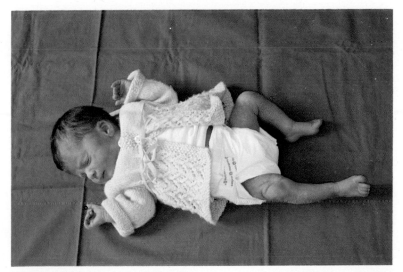

Fig. 32 Asymmetric tonic neck reflex.

1 | Normal Infant and Examination (12)

Care of the full-term infant

Birth
If the baby is in good condition, he can be given immediately to the parents for them to hold and inspect. Some babies do not breathe by 2 min and need ventilation by intubation or bag and mask. Any meconium must be aspirated carefully from the respiratory tract.

Warmth
Hypothermia can easily occur and may cause further complications. The baby must be dried carefully and then wrapped and kept in a warm environment (Fig. 33). The infant's temperature should be measured on admission to the postnatal ward.

Feeding
There is a definite advantage in breast feeding (Fig. 34) and this should begin in the labour ward. Supplements of artificial milk should be strongly discouraged, especially if there is a family history of allergy.

Infection
Newborn babies are easily colonised with pathogenic organisms. All staff must pay particular attention to handwashing between touching babies. The umbilical cord is a favourite site for colonisation; it should be left uncovered and treated with alcohol only.

Family relationships
The baby should not be taken away from the mother unless absolutely necessary, and should be nursed next to the mother's bed. Everyone who works in a maternity hospital should do their best to discourage any practice which interferes with the normal relationship of a mother and her baby.

Examination
A full medical examination of the infant should be done within 24 h of birth to exclude major congenital abnormalities and to reassure the parents that the baby is well.

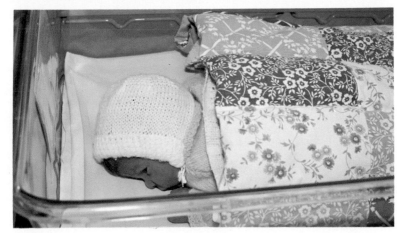

Fig. 33 Baby should be kept well wrapped and in warm environment to prevent hypothermia.

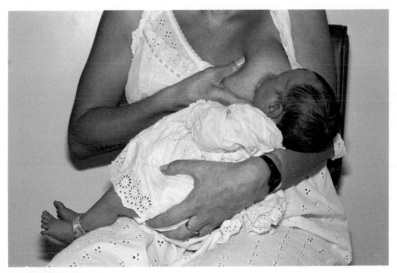

Fig. 34 Breast feeding.

Birth Trauma and Postural Defects (1)

Moulding of the head

Clinical features

Elongation and narrowing of the skull (Fig. 35) with overlapping of cranial sutures occurs as part of the normal birth process in most vaginal deliveries.

Course and prognosis

Normal shape of the head returns within a few days of birth.

Caput succedaneum

Clinical features

Subcutaneous oedema and bruising of the presenting part (Fig. 36), usually the parietal or occipital region of the head.

Course and prognosis

The swelling is maximal immediately after birth, and disappears spontaneously within a few days.

Cephalhaematoma

Incidence

Less common than caput, but still common.

Clinical features

Cephalhaematoma occurs from rupture of small vessels in the periosteum. There is a soft swelling or lump, often the size and shape of a table tennis ball, with a very discrete edge (Figs 37 & 38). They occur over the presenting part, usually the parietal bone, are sometimes bilateral and are often associated with caput. By contrast with caput, cephalhaematomas are not apparent at birth, but there is a gradual ooze of blood from small vessel rupture, causing a slow increase to maximal size within a few days of birth. The swelling never crosses a suture.

Course and prognosis

They disappear spontaneously, sometimes accompanied by calcification, but may take several weeks or months to completely resolve. Jaundice is a common complication in the first few weeks.

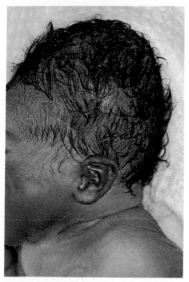

Fig. 35 Moulding and caput in vertex presentation.

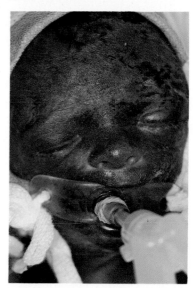

Fig. 36 Bruising of the face after face presentation.

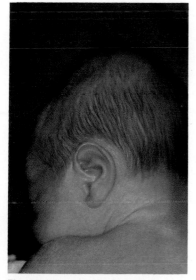

Fig. 37 Lateral view of parietal cephalhaematoma.

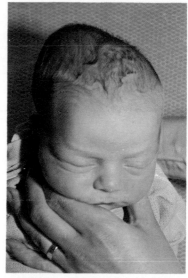

Fig. 38 Parietal cephalhaematoma.

Birth Trauma and Postural Defects (2)

Postural deformities

Incidence

Postural and compressional effects occur frequently. The majority are mild and transient.

Clinical features

With abnormal presentations, the intra-uterine posture is often maintained for several days after birth.

After a face or brow presentation, the infant may lie with head and neck extended in an opisthotonic posture.

After breech delivery, the head is not moulded like that of a baby after vertex delivery. The legs are often maintained in hip flexion for some days (Figs 39 & 40). In many normal infants, the feet are often moulded into postural talipes (Fig. 41). Postural talipes can always be fully reduced by passive manipulation and there is a full range of foot and ankle movement.

Extensive bruising of the presenting part often occurs, particularly if there has been an abnormal presentation. It resolves gradually over a few days and is often accompanied by hyperbilirubinaemia.

Course and prognosis

After abnormal presentations, postural deformities disappear rapidly spontaneously. Postural talipes may take months to completely resolve.

Management

No special management is required as all improve spontaneously. Passive manipulation or even splinting of the feet is sometimes advised for postural talipes, but there is no evidence that it hastens the normal resolution.

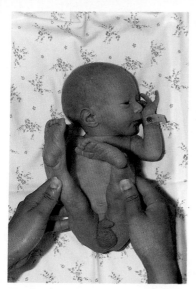

Fig. 39 Extended breech position.

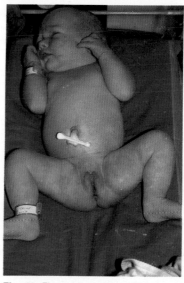

Fig. 40 Flexed breech position.

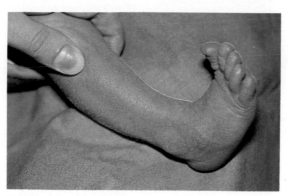

Fig. 41 Postural talipes.

Birth Trauma and Postural Defects (3)

Facial palsy

Incidence
Common.

Aetiology
Compression of the facial nerve as it exits from the parotid gland, sometimes caused by pressure from forceps blades, but often occurs after normal vaginal delivery.

Clinical features
Weakness, usually unilateral, of the facial muscles (Fig. 42) which may cause drooping of the mouth (Fig. 43) and sometimes dribbling. There is often feeding difficulty and inability to close the eye on the affected side.

Prognosis
Majority resolve spontaneously within a few days or weeks after birth.

Erb's palsy

Incidence
Uncommon.

Aetiology
Stretching or tearing of the upper part of the brachial plexus, usually caused by neck traction during breech delivery or with shoulder dystocia.

Clinical features
The affected arm and hand assume the waiter's tip position (Fig. 44)—weakness or paralysis of abduction at the shoulder, with flexion at the elbow and extension and supination of the wrist.

Prognosis
The weakness or paralysis usually responds spontaneously over a period of weeks or months, but paralysis occasionally is permanent. If resolution takes a long time, passive physiotherapy and night splints will prevent the formation of contractures.

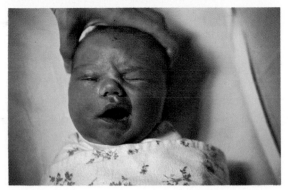

Fig. 42 Facial palsy after face presentation.

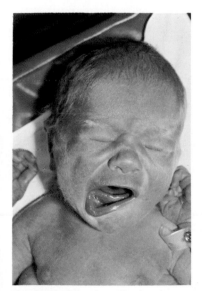

Fig. 43 Facial palsy affecting the lower lip.

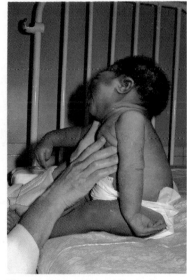

Fig. 44 Erb's palsy with arm in waiter's tip position.

2 | Birth Trauma and Postural Defects (4)

Obstetric manipulations

Incidence

Obstetric manipulations often cause unavoidable, trivial skin trauma. With careful application and removal of instruments and equipment, they can usually be kept to a minimum.

Clinical features

Forceps application often results in pressure indentation or bruising (Fig. 45) and occasionally causes facial palsy or subcutaneous fat necrosis. Both of these complications can also occur after a spontaneous vaginal delivery, particularly after a long labour with slow descent of the presenting part. Subcutaneous fat necrosis can occur (Fig. 46) over any bony prominence, but is most common on the cheek. It usually presents as an indurated, sometimes red, area which may then develop necrosis with loss of subcutaneous fat and sometimes calcification.

Artificial rupture of the membranes, fetal scalp sampling and scalp electrodes may all cause incised wounds (Fig. 47). Particular care should be taken when removing scalp clips, as incorrect detachment may result in a core of scalp being removed.

Ventouse extraction, by applying suction to the scalp to assist delivery when there is delay in the second stage of labour, frequently causes bruising and a chignon-shaped caput. Sometimes it causes more serious blistering, abrasions or laceration of the presenting part (Fig. 48), or occasionally subaponeurotic haemorrhage.

Significance

Lesions are usually trivial, but may become the site of infection.

Course and prognosis

Most resolve spontaneously without significant scarring or more permanent sequelae.

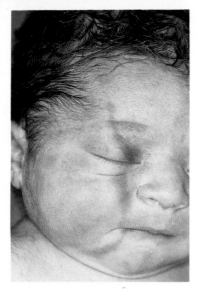

Fig. 45 Forceps mark.

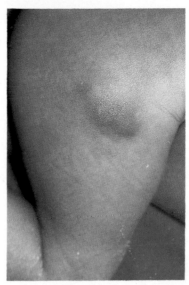

Fig. 46 Red indurated area of sub-cutaneous fat necrosis on thigh.

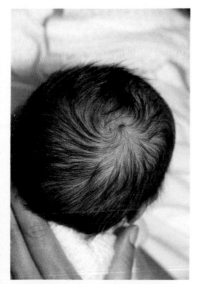

Fig. 47 Wound from a scalp clip used for fetal heart monitoring.

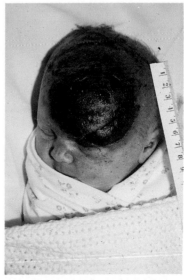

Fig. 48 Very severe abrasion from a prolonged application of ventouse.

3 | Iatrogenic Lesions (1)

Skin lesions

Incidence

With increasing use and complexity of neonatal intensive care, iatrogenic lesions, particularly of the skin, are becoming common.

Aetiology and clinical features

Traumatic abrasions of the skin occur frequently, particularly in very preterm infants (Fig. 49) and may be associated with the use of adhesive plaster, name bands or starched sheets. Radiant heaters increase insensitive water loss through the transparent skin of preterm infants and may cause drying and fragility of the skin. Transcutaneous skin monitors for measuring O_2 and CO_2 always leave a transient, superficial, pink burn which does not usually cause scarring unless the electrode has been left in situ for a prolonged period. Depigmented circular areas of skin are sometimes seen later in coloured infants (Fig. 50). Invasive procedures such as intercostal catheters for draining pneumothoraces (Fig. 51), radial artery puncture and repeated heel pricking may leave scars. Intercostal catheters should be sited carefully, avoiding the breast bud in order to avoid more serious damage to the breast in later life.

Management and prevention

Measures should be taken to avoid excessive use of adhesive plasters or equipment whenever possible.
Protective covering may limit insensible water loss by evaporation in the days immediately after birth, but will obviously depend on whether the clinical condition of the infant allows such covering. After the early days or weeks of life, the skin becomes much thicker and less prone to traumatic damage, even in very immature infants.

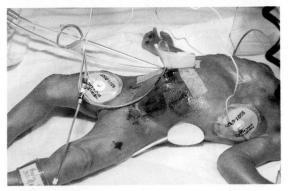

Fig. 49 Skin abrasions from adhesive tape.

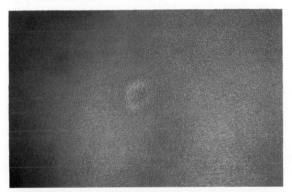

Fig. 50 Depigmented areas from transcutaneous electrode.

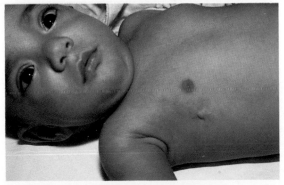

Fig. 51 Scar from a drain for pneumothorax.

Catheter and infusion complications

Clinical features and aetiology

Catheters in major vessels may cause obstruction and ischaemic necrosis to distal extremities, thrombosis or embolism. Such complications are uncommon. Transient cyanosis of the leg is sometimes seen after insertion of an umbilical arterial catheter, and if it does not resolve rapidly or if there is associated pallor or absence of arterial pulses, the catheter should be removed immediately. Cyanosis of the toes, particularly after arterial infusion is commenced, is not uncommon. It is usually transient and associated with minor air embolism.

With prolonged catheterisation, the risk of infection and necrotising enterocolitis increases. Peripheral intravenous infusion sites are often associated with oedema or extravasation of the infusion fluid when the drip tissues. Infusions containing irritants such as calcium or sodium bicarbonate may cause serious tissue necrosis (Fig. 52) and lead to ulceration and later scar formation (Figs 53 & 54).

Management and prevention

Care should be taken in siting peripheral infusions to avoid veins near joints. Scarring around joints may cause contractures later. All intravenous drips should be checked frequently to ensure that they are running into the vein, particularly when infusion pumps are used. Central catheters should always be removed if there is persistent cyanosis of the extremities, or if there are signs of catheter occlusion or impaired circulation to the limbs, kidneys or gut. Arterial catheters should be removed as soon as the infant's clinical condition improves and when sampling for blood gas analysis is required less often.

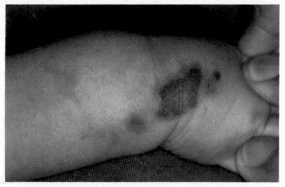

Fig. 52 Recent subcutaneous extravasation of fluid.

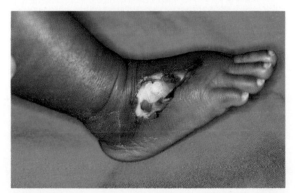

Fig. 53 Ulceration after extravasation of an irritant fluid.

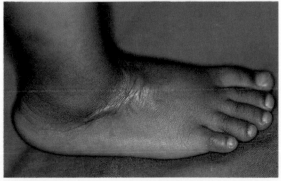

Fig. 54 A scar after an ulcer had healed.

4 | Skin Disorders (1)

Strawberry naevi

Incidence

Common, particularly in preterm infants.

Pathology

Dilated capillaries with or without endothelial proliferation.

Clinical features

Raised, soft, pitted, bright red haemangiomata with a discrete edge. They are usually not present at birth, but appear within the first few weeks of life. They are often preceded by a small, slightly raised, bright red spot, which evolves into the strawberry naevus (Fig. 55). They may be single or multiple and occur anywhere on the body.

Course and prognosis

The majority increase rapidly in size during the first year of life. Ulceration and subsequent infection may occur in the centre of the lesion. All strawberry naevi regress slowly over the next years. Involution has started when pale grey areas of fibrosis appear in the centre of the naevus (Fig. 56). They eventually disappear completely (Fig. 57) and leave only a flat, pale depigmented area.

Management

No treatment is required, unless there is repeated haemorrhage, infection or severe cosmetic deformity interfering with function of the affected part. All forms of treatment except steroids will leave some scarring of the skin; natural resolution is the optimal management in the majority of strawberry naevi.

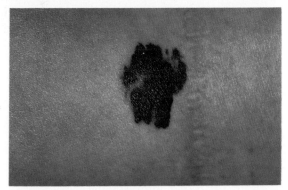

Fig. 55 Early strawberry naevus.

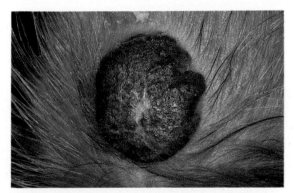

Fig. 56 Strawberry naevus beginning to regress.

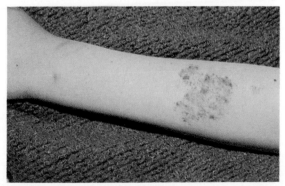

Fig. 57 Fading strawberry naevus.

4 | Skin Disorders (2)

Port wine stains

Synonym
Naevus flammeus.

Clinical features
Sharply demarcated flat capillary haemangiomata which may vary in colour from pale pink to deep purple (Fig. 58). They are present at birth and do not increase in size after birth. They may occur anywhere on the body, but are most common on the face.

Course and prognosis
The majority remain as a permanent discoloration of the skin.

Associations
Most port wine stains occur as an isolated defect but sometimes are partly cavernous, involve other organs or form part of a recognisable vascular syndrome, e.g. Sturge–Weber syndrome (Fig. 59).

Management
Generally, surgery is cosmetically unsatisfactory. The use of a cosmetic cover-up cream may be helpful in older children.

Cavernous hamangiomata

Pathology
Large, dilated blood-filled cavities with venous anastamoses. There is often a surface capillary element.

Clinical features
Soft, subcutaneous bluish-red mass (Fig. 60) with a less distinct edge than a strawberry naevus.

Course and prognosis
The majority do not regress with age and may actually increase in size. Haemorrhage and infection sometimes occur, and occasionally sequestration of platelets within the naevus may cause thrombocytopenia.

Management
Surgical excision is often difficult. Injection of sclerosing agents under anaesthetic may promote fibrosis and eventual diminution in size.

NEONATOLOGY

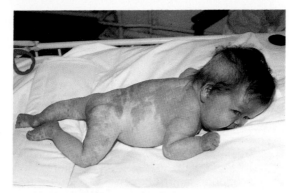

Fig. 58 Extensive port wine stain.

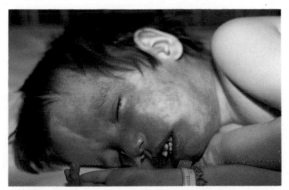

Fig. 59 Facial naevus of Sturge–Weber syndrome.

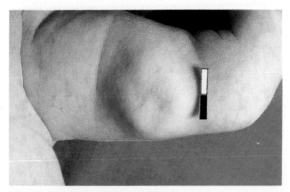

Fig. 60 Cavernous haemangioma.

4 | Skin Disorders (3)

Pigmented and depigmented naevi

Incidence

Uncommon in the neonatal period with the exception of Mongolian blue spots.

Clinical features

Small localised pigmented naevi are of no clinical significance. Severe cosmetic deformity may occur with the rare giant bathing trunk naevus. Incontinentia pigmenti, a rare sex-linked hereditary disorder, initially consists of inflammatory bullae in the neonatal period which progress to pigmented streaks in the later stages of the disease (Fig. 61).
Depigmented lesions are also uncommon and may occur as an isolated finding (Fig. 62). Occasionally, areas of skin or hair depigmentation may be the only manifestation of tuberose sclerosis in the neonatal period.

Management

Depends on the cosmetic deformity and presence or absence of associated disorders. Giant bathing trunk naevi are often grossly disfiguring and may be improved with multiple tiny skin grafts.

Partial thickness skin defects

Incidence

Rare.

Aetiology

Unknown.

Clinical features

The lesion is usually a superficial area of ulceration, most commonly found on the scalp.

Association

Partial thickness skin defects of the scalp sometimes occur in trisomy 13 (Patau's syndrome—Fig. 63).

Course and prognosis

The defect heals by granulation. If it is not superficial, or if secondary infection occurs, healing may result in scar formation and contraction. A permanent bald patch may be left on the scalp.

NEONATOLOGY

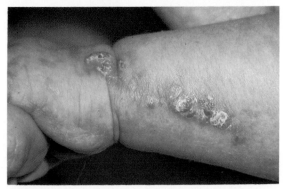

Fig. 61 Lesions of incontinentia pigmenti in a linear distribution.

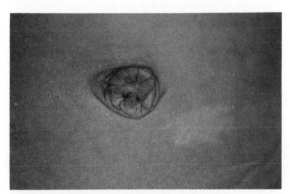

Fig. 62 Depigmented lesion alongside the umbilicus in a normal infant.

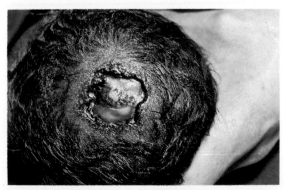

Fig. 63 Scalp skin defect in trisomy 13.

Epidermolysis bullosa letalis

Incidence
Very rare.

Inheritance
Autosomal recessive.

Pathology
Subepidermal bullae with blisters between the basement membrane of the epidermis and the connective tissue of the dermis.

Clinical features
Bullae present at or soon after birth and cover large areas of the body. The bullae characteristically appear after minor trauma (Figs 64 & 65).

Differential diagnosis
There are several different varieties of epidermolysis bullosa. Those which appear in later infancy are usually autosomal dominant, and often dystrophic resulting in scar formation. Epidermolysis bullosa may be similar in appearance to widespread staphylococcal skin infection (pemphigus neonatorum or toxic epidermal necrolysis) (Fig. 66), but should be differentiated by culture.

Management
Good nursing care with particular emphasis on minimal handling because of the dramatic effect of minor trauma on the skin.
Antibiotics may be required if there is secondary bacterial infection.

Prognosis
High mortality in the neonatal form.

Antenatal diagnosis
A fetal skin biopsy in the second trimester may be helpful in high-risk pregnancies when there has been a previously affected infant.

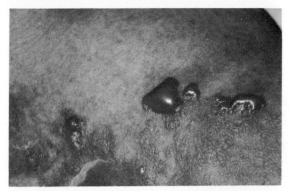

Fig. 64 Typical bullae of epidermolysis bullosa.

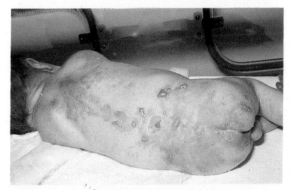

Fig. 65 Widespread bullae.

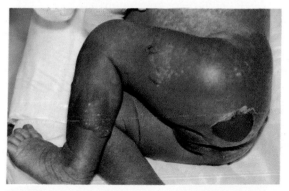

Fig. 66 Bullae may be similar in appearance to toxic epidermal necrolysis.

Collodion baby

Incidence

Very rare.

Aetiology

Unknown.

Clinical features

At birth, the infant is encased in a shiny, brownish-yellow, cellophane-like membrane (Figs 67 & 68) which may be taut and may distort the facial features and extremities. Respiratory embarrassment may occur because of restriction of chest expansion. A similar, but more severe, condition is the harlequin fetus where there are deep fissures between scale-like areas of skin. Ectropion and fish-mouth also occur in the harlequin fetus (Figs 69 & 70). The harlequin vascular phenomenon is a quite different condition.

Course and prognosis

Desquamation of the membranous skin occurs after birth and may take several months to be complete. There is no particular treatment. The skin should not be allowed to become too dry and secondary infection should be treated promptly. Prognosis should be guarded for collodion babies, because although most have normal skin in later childhood, a few develop ichthyotic skin changes later. The harlequin fetus invariably dies in the neonatal period.

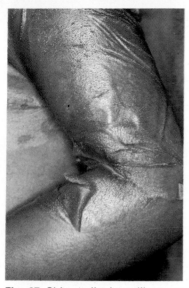

Fig. 67 Shiny cellophane-like membrane of collodion baby.

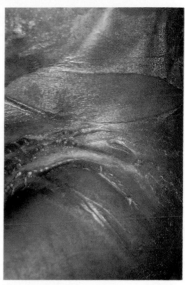

Fig. 68 Desquamating membrane.

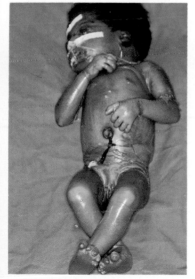

Fig. 69 Harlequin fetus.

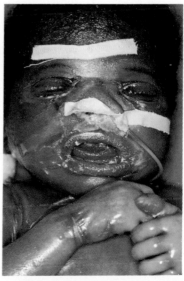

Fig. 70 Ectropion and fish-mouth of harlequin fetus.

Accessory skin tags and polydactyly

Incidence
Common, particularly in negro infants.

Inheritance
Usually autosomal dominant.

Clinical features
Accessory skin tags (accessory auricles) often occur on the face, anterior to the ear (Fig. 71) Accessory nipples (Fig. 72) are often mistaken for pigmented naevi. They may be single or multiple and usually occur in a direct line beneath the normally situated nipple.
Extra digits (polydactyly) vary in appearance from loosely attached skin tags to fully-formed fingers or toes (Fig. 73). They are usually attached at the base of the normal little finger or toe.
Occasionally there may be an associated bifid metacarpal or metatarsal bone.

Significance
Usually only a cosmetic deformity, but extra toes may cause broadening of the forefoot with difficulty in fitting shoes later.

Management
Small pedunculated tags can be ligated if the pedicle and base is very narrow and does not contain cartilage. The tag will become ischaemic but it is not painful. It will usually separate from the base within a few days leaving a small dry scar. If the base is broad or if the tag has a cartilaginous attachment, plastic surgery will be required.

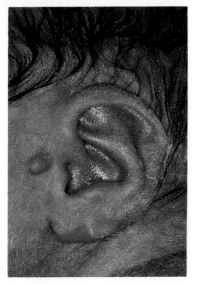

Fig. 71 Accessory auricle.

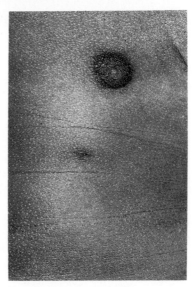

Fig. 72 Accessory nipple.

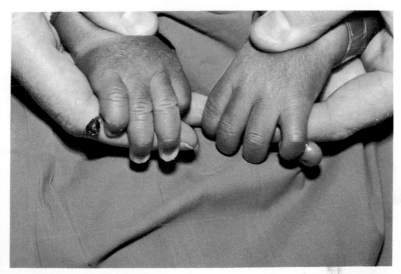

Fig. 73 Bilateral polydactyly.

Talipes equino varus

Synonym	Club foot.
Incidence	1 in 1000 live births. Twice as common in males as in females.
Aetiology	Uncertain; probably polygenic inheritance and intra-uterine pressure play a part.
Clinical features	The affected foot is held in a fixed flexion (equinus) and inturned (varus) position (Fig. 74). It can be differentiated from positional talipes because the deformity in true talipes cannot be passively corrected.
Associations	Usually occurs as an isolated deformity but may occur in association with meningomyelocele, oligohydramnios, congenital dislocation of the hip.
Management	Correction of the deformity is usually initially attempted by splinting; but if correction is difficult, surgical release of the contracted structures in the calf and ankle may be necessary.

Toe deformities

Incidence	Common—particularly syndactyly.
Inheritance	Mostly autosomal dominant.
Clinical features	Syndactyly usually occurs as webbing of the second and third toes. Overlapping of the little toe over the fourth toe is usually bilateral (Fig. 75). Hammer toe usually occurs in the big toe and results from a congenital contracture of the flexor tendons (Fig. 76).
Management	Syndactyly of toes does not require surgery. The position of the toes in hammer toe or overlapping little toe is usually uncomfortable and surgical correction may be needed.

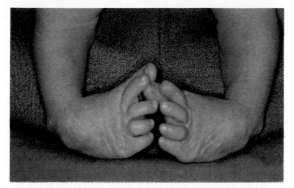

Fig. 74 Bilateral talipes equino varus.

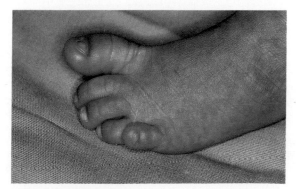

Fig. 75 Over-riding little toe.

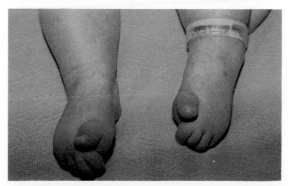

Fig. 76 Bilateral hammer toes.

5 | Congenital Abnormalities (3)

Neural tube defects

Synonyms

Meningomyelocele, spina bifida; encephalocele; anencephaly.

Incidence

Varies in different geographical locations. It is particularly common in the USA and UK where the overall incidence of neural tube defects is 1 in 300 pregnancies. Neural tube defects are more common in the Welsh and Irish than in the English. The high birth prevalence is falling for reasons which are not yet clear, but may be related to antenatal screening with ultrasound and alpha fetoprotein, and improved maternal nutrition. Spina bifida occulta occurs in at least 1% of the normal population.

Aetiology

Unknown; but there has been much speculation about the role of nutritional deficiencies.

Inheritance

Polygenic; after one affected child, there is a 1 in 20 risk of recurrence of a neural tube defect in the next pregnancy.

Antenatal diagnosis

Elevated alpha fetoprotein concentrations in amniotic fluid and maternal plasma occur in the second trimester of pregnancy in the majority of open neural tube defects. Spinal defects are usually apparent on ultrasound examination.

Meningomyelocele and meningocele

Clinical features

A fluid-filled sac often containing neural tissue, meningomyelocele, with an underlying defect of the spinal arch occurs in the lumbo-sacral region (Figs 77 & 78) in 94% of cases. The degree of handicap depends on the level and severity of the defect. There may be flaccid paralysis of the lower limbs, sensory loss, a neurogenic bladder with urinary incontinence, and a patulous anus (Fig. 79) with faecal incontinence. Meningoceles often occur in the thoracic (Fig. 80) or cervical spine.

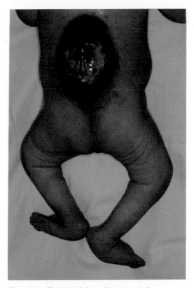

Fig. 77 Typical lumbo-sacral meningomyelocele.

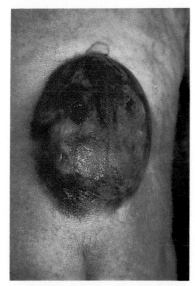

Fig. 78 Meningomyelocele with exposed nervous tissue.

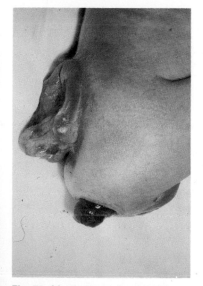

Fig. 79 Meningomyelocele with paralysed anus. There is a rectal prolapse.

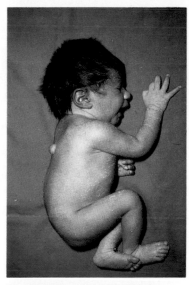

Fig. 80 Thoracic meningocele.

Meningomyelocele and meningocele
(contd)

Associations

Hydrocephalus occurs in 70% of cases of meningomyelocele. Congenital dislocation of the hip, and talipes equino varus are common, and urinary tract infections often occur.

Management

Surgery may be indicated in less severely handicapped infants after careful assessment of the congenital abnormalities and neurological state of the infant in the first few days of life. Skin closure is the first operation, but many other surgical procedures may be required to treat hydrocephalus, orthopaedic and urinary problems. The meningoceles in the thoracic or cervical regions usually have an excellent prognosis as there are no associated neurological abnormalities.

Encephalocele

Clinical features

Herniation of the meninges and brain through the skull (Fig. 81).

Course and prognosis

Depends on the amount of brain which has to be excised in order to close the skull defect, but the prognosis is not necessarily poor. The lesions are usually occipital.

Anencephaly

Clinical features

Absence of the forebrain and skull vault, and secondary distortion of the face and ears (Fig. 82).

Associations

Other abnormalities are common, particularly cleft palate and abnormal cervical vertebrae. It is commoner in females.

Course and prognosis

Anencephaly is incompatible with life. Many infants are stillborn, although a few may survive for several hours and occasionally days.

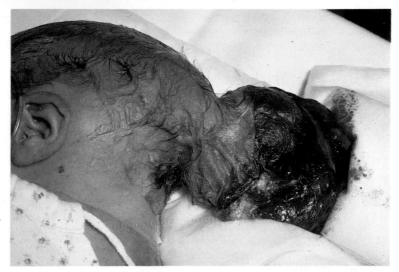

Fig. 81 Occipital encephalocele.

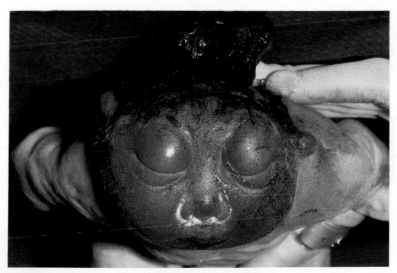

Fig. 82 Anencephaly. (By courtesy of Dr Gillian Gau.)

Hydrocephalus

Aetiology

May occur as an isolated congenital abnormality. Most commonly due to aqueduct stenosis, or secondary to intraventricular haemorrhage or neonatal meningitis. It is commonly found in association with neural tube defects.

Clinical features

Accelerated rate of growth of the skull gives rise to enlargement of the head circumference (Fig. 83), widening of the fontanelles and sutures. When severe and untreated, hydrocephalus may give rise to a setting-sun apearance of the eyes, mental handicap and upper motor neurone signs, particularly in the legs.

Management

Depends on aetiology and severity. Ultrasound and CT scan will confirm the diagnosis. If there is evidence of continuing deviation from the normal rate of growth of the ventricles or skull circumference, a ventriculo-peritoneal or ventriculo-atrial shunt may be required.

Course and prognosis

Not all infants with hydrocephalus require neurosurgery. After intraventricular haemorrhage, hydrocephalus may be transient and limited by serial lumbar puncture. Following shunt surgery, the prognosis depends on the underlying aetiology, extent of preceding brain damage and the occurrence of shunt complications.

Microcephaly

Clinical features

Head circumference below the 3rd centile for age and gestation (Fig. 84), and which is inappropriately small for the length and weight of the infant.

Aetiology

Usually unknown; often associated with mental retardation. Sometimes a clear prenatal cause is known, e.g. congenital rubella or cytomegalovirus infection.

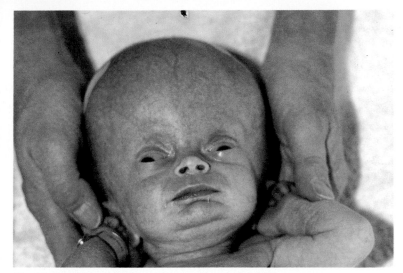

Fig. 83 Hydrocephalus.

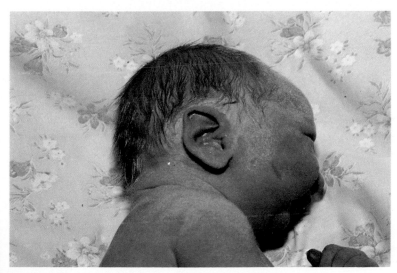

Fig. 84 Microcephaly.

Cleft lip and palate

Incidence

Common; approx. 1 in 600 live births. More frequent in East Asia.

Inheritance

Familial; no simple Mendelian pattern. Probably polygenic inheritance.

Clinical features

Isolated clefts of the palate always occur in the midline. The least obvious type is the submucous cleft which is often associated with a bifid uvula. Cleft lip and palate may be unilateral (Fig. 85) or bilateral (Fig. 86).

Associations

Feeding difficulties and orthodontic deformities are common. Speech problems may occur with cleft palate, particularly after late closure. Deafness may arise secondary to regurgitation and sepsis in the nasopharynx.

Management

Some infants can feed from the breast; most infants feed well through a large teat. Tube or spoon feeding may occasionally be needed. Surgery is performed in several stages. Repair of the cleft lip to correct the cosmetic deformity should be performed as soon as possible after birth. The palate repair is usually done later, but within the first year of life. If the initial deformity is severe, secondary repair of the lip or nose, or pharyngoplasty may be required in later childhood.

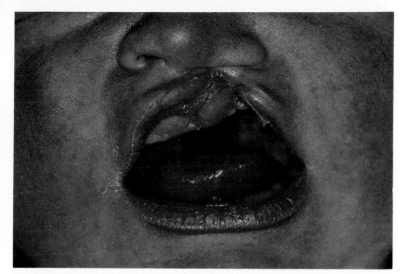

Fig. 85 Unilateral cleft lip with cleft palate.

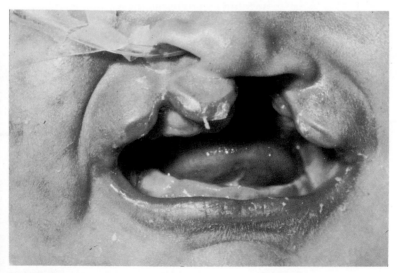

Fig. 86 Bilateral cleft lip with cleft palate.

Cataracts

Incidence
Uncommon.

Aetiology
Congenital cataracts are often inherited as an autosomal dominant. They may also occur secondary to intra-uterine infections, particularly rubella, or metabolic disorders such as galactosaemia.

Clinical features
An opaque mass can be seen in the pupil (Fig. 87).

Management
Depends on the type and severity of the cataract, and the interference with vision. Metabolic disorders, which may be potentially treatable, should always be excluded. Early surgery is indicated within the first month of life in those cataracts which warrant treatment. After surgery for cataracts at any age, contact lenses will need to be fitted and replaced at regular intervals.

Cystic hygroma

Incidence
Uncommon.

Aetiology
Hamartoma of the jugular lymphatic vessels.

Clinical features
Soft, multi-cystic, ill-defined fluctuant lymphatic swelling in the lateral part of the neck (Fig. 88). The cysts transilluminate well and enlarge slowly during the first few months or years of life. The effect on the child depends on the size and site of the abnormality, but can occasionally cause dysphagia or respiratory obstruction, particularly if it enlarges rapidly. Occasionally enlargement may be due to infection or haemorrhage.

Management
Surgical excision is difficult because of the invasive, ill-defined nature of the lymphatic channels, but it is usually necessary.

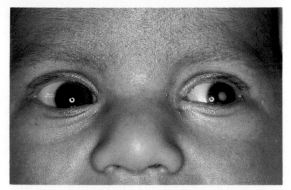

Fig. 87 Unilateral congenital cataract.

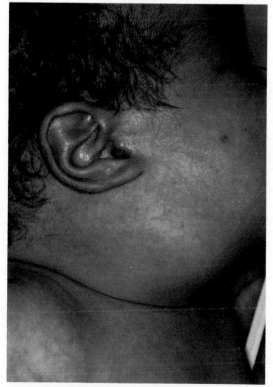

Fig. 88 Cystic hygroma.

Congenital dislocation of the hip

Incidence

Dislocated or dislocatible hip at birth may be as common as 1 in 100 live births. With early detection and treatment, the prevalence of dislocated hip after the first year of life has been reduced from 1 : 1000 to 1 : 10000. It is commoner in girls and after breech presentation.

Inheritance

Familial; no simple Mendelian pattern of inheritance.

Clinical features

The majority should be detected by routine screening tests in the neonatal period. Fixed dislocation can be diagnosed by finding restricted abduction of the hip and sometimes shortening of the affected leg.

To examine for a reducible dislocation, the infant should be placed on his back on a firm surface. Holding the thighs between finger and thumb with the hips and knees both flexed, each hip should be slowly abducted through 90° starting from the midline (Figs 89, 90 & 91). A palpable 'clunk' will be felt as a posteriorly dislocated hip slips back into the acetabulum. A gentle attempt should then be made to diagnose a dislocatible hip. With the leg adducted, pressure is applied with the thumb on the upper part of the femur; the leg is then abducted, as above.

Management

Abduction splinting is required for at least 6 weeks. Even a dislocatible hip which resolves spontaneously should be observed until the child is walking. X-ray all hips where neonatal examinations have aroused suspicion at 4–6 months of age. Delay in diagnosis may involve more prolonged splinting or surgery. With early diagnosis and treatment, the majority of infants with congenital dislocation of the hip should have no delay in crawling or walking.

NEONATOLOGY

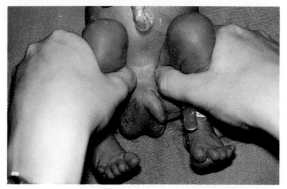

Fig. 89 Examination of the hips starting in the midline with hips and knees flexed.

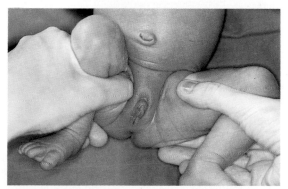

Fig. 90 Abduction of the hip holding the thigh between fingers and thumb.

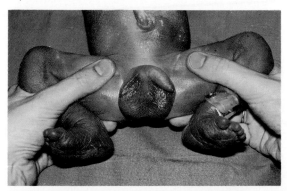

Fig. 91 Full abduction of both hips through 90°.

Congenital heart disease

Incidence

7 in 1 000 live births; high incidence in infants of diabetic mothers and infants with chromosomal abnormalities.

Clinical features

Most present with a heart murmur, cardiac failure or cyanosis (Fig. 92); they may become breathless and sweat with feeds, and usually fail to thrive.

Management

After careful clinical examination, a chest X-ray and ECG may be helpful in the assessment. Echocardiography or cardiac catheterisation may be necessary for precise diagnosis.

Oesophageal atresia and tracheo-oesophageal fistula (TOF)

Incidence

1 in 3 000 live births.

Clinical features

Excessive accumulation of saliva and mucus in the mouth and pharynx occurs because there is a developmental anomaly with a blind-ending upper oesophageal pouch. Respiratory distress may occur if there is spill-over into the trachea or regurgitation of stomach contents through a fistula. Pulmonary complications frequently occur if the baby is fed before the diagnosis is suspected.

Associations

Maternal hydramnios occurs in 60% babies with oesophageal atresia. When hydramnios is present, a firm catheter should be passed to test for gastric acid.

Diagnosis

Chest X-ray will usually confirm oesophageal atresia (Fig. 93). Air in the stomach indicates the presence of a fistula.

Management

Early surgery with primary anastamosis if possible. Fistulae should be sought and ligated.

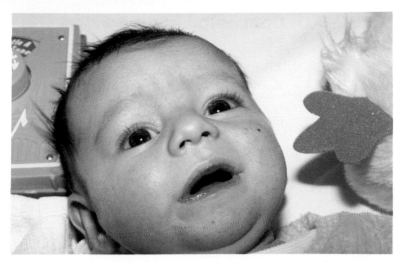

Fig. 92 Central cyanosis.

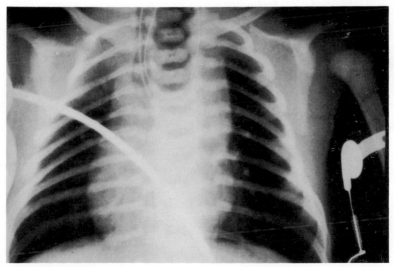

Fig. 93 X-ray showing oesophageal atresia.

Amniotic bands and amputations

Incidence

Uncommon, but exact incidence is not known. Clustering of cases has been reported.

Aetiology

Unknown; the most widely accepted hypothesis suggests that the developing embryo may lie in a false cavity between the amnion and chorion after traumatic rupture of the amnion in the first trimester. The membranes may then form encircling bands around the limbs. An alternative hypothesis is that vascular occlusion secondary to embolisation from thrombosed placental vessels may cause the abnormalities.

Associations

Amniotic bands may be associated with fetal malformations, particularly limb or cranio-facial defects.

Clinical features

The presence of amniotic bands is usually inferred when constriction rings (Fig. 94) or reduction deformities of the limbs occur (Fig. 95). Occasionally a band may be attached to the fetus at the site of a local abnormality.

Limb reduction deformities

Aetiology

A famous outbreak in the early 1960s was due to the effects of a teratogen—thalidomide. Many cases occur without any known cause.

Clinical features

The lesion is obvious at birth. The limb is short and a rudimentary hand or foot may be attached to the shoulder or hip.

Management

A search should be made for other abnormalities. The baby is referred to a limb-fitting centre in early life.

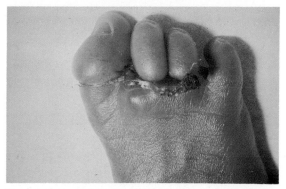

Fig. 94 Constriction ring around toes.

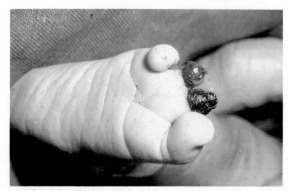

Fig. 95 Amputation of toes.

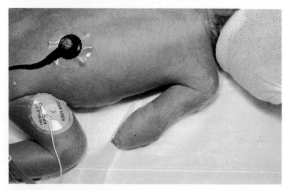

Fig. 96 Arm reduction deformity with vestigial fingers.

Syndromes (1)

Down's syndrome

Synonyms	Trisomy 21, mongolism.
Incidence	1 in 600 live births; the most common chromosomal abnormality.
Inheritance	Increased incidence of trisomy 21 with older maternal age (1 in 100 live births after maternal age of 40 years and 1 in 50, over 45 years). General risk of recurrence is 1%, but may be higher if there is translocation and, for older mothers, is the expected incidence for maternal age.
Aetiology	Trisomy 21 occurs in 94% infants, translocation in 3% and mosaicism in 3%.
Clinical features	Low birth weight and growth retardation are common. Mongoloid facies (Figs 97 & 98), generalised hypotonia, brachycephaly with a flattened occiput, a third fontanelle and single transverse palmar creases (Simian crease—Fig. 99) are usually present. There may also be incurving of short fifth finger, a wide gap between second and third toe, marked plantar crease, congenital heart disease and Brushfield's spots.
Associations	Increased incidence of respiratory infection, leukaemia, thyroid disease, duodenal atresia and Hirschsprung's disease.
Course and prognosis	Short stature and mental retardation are always present. Average IQ is less than 50, although social performance is often beyond that expected for mental age. Males are invariably infertile, but females are not necessarily so. Average life span is 30–40 years.
Antenatal diagnosis	Amniocentesis and chromosomal analysis may be indicated in older mothers, or when there has been a previously affected child, and when there is a translocation.

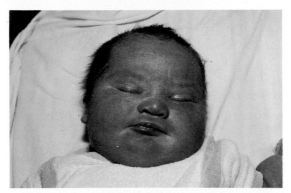

Fig. 97 Typical mongoloid facies.

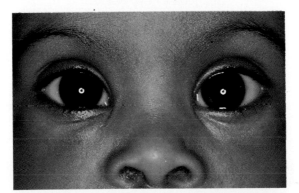

Fig. 98 Prominent epicanthic folds in Down's syndrome.

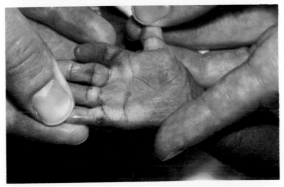

Fig. 99 Single transverse palmar crease (Simian crease).

Edward's syndrome

Synonyms	Trisomy 18, E-trisomy.
Incidence	Occurs in 1 in 3 000 live births; second most common chromosomal abnormality.
Inheritance	Recurrence risk is low.
Clinical features	Small for gestational age. Severe mental retardation. Hypoplastic lungs. Congenital heart disease. Abnormal posture with flexion deformities of hips and limbs (Fig. 100). Clenched hands with overlapping of index finger over third, and fifth finger over fourth finger (Fig. 101). Rocker-bottom feet (Fig. 102). Renal abnormalities and cryptorchidism. Cranio-facial abnormalities with prominent occiput, micrognathia, hirsutism, short palpebral fissures, microstomia, facial palsy and low-set ears.
Course and prognosis	Majority die within first few months of life. Less than 10% survive longer than 1 year.

Patau's syndrome

Synonym	Trisomy 13, D-trisomy.
Inheritance	Recurrence risk is low.
Clinical features	Midline defects of face, eyes and forebrain. Cleft lip and palate. Severe mental retardation. Deafness. Rocker-bottom feet (Fig. 102). Congenital heart defects. Cryptorchidism.
Course and prognosis	Less than 20% survive the first year of life.

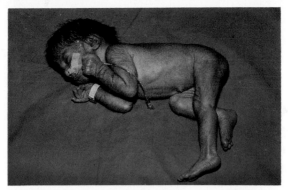

Fig. 100 Edward's syndrome with typical flexion deformities of hips and limbs.

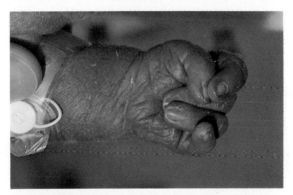

Fig. 101 Clenched hands with overlapping of fingers in Edward's syndrome.

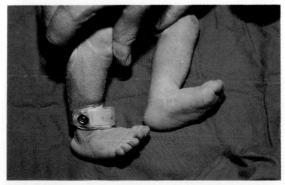

Fig. 102 Rocker-bottom feet.

6 | Syndromes (3)

Turner's syndrome

Synonyms	XO syndrome, single X syndrome.
Incidence	1 in 5 000 live births.
Inheritance	Usually sporadic occurrence.
Aetiology	Premature ovarian failure. Single X chromosome and absence of sex chromatin.
Clinical features	Low birth weight, female infants with transient congenital lymphoedema of hands and feet (Fig. 103). Webbing of neck, broad chest with widely-spaced nipples, low hairline and short neck and a wide carrying angle (cubitus valgus).
Associations	Coarctation of aorta, deafness and mild mental deficiency occur in about 10%.
Course and prognosis	Short stature and failure of secondary sexual development become apparent in later childhood.
Management	Cyclical oestrogen replacement therapy will be indicated during adolescence and adult life to induce development of secondary sexual characteristics. Infertility is invariable.

Short-limbed dwarfism

Synonym	Chondrodysplasia.
Incidence	Achondroplasia, the most common chondrodysplasia occurs in 1 in 10 000 live births.
Inheritance	Autosomal dominant inheritance; approximately 90% occur as a fresh mutation. The lethal forms of chondrodysplasia (asphyxiating thoracic dystrophy or thanatophoric dwarfism) are usually autosomal recessive (Fig. 104).
Clinical features	Short limbs, a large head (macrocephaly) and a prominent forehead with a broad nasal bridge.
Course and prognosis	Intelligence is usually normal in achondroplastic dwarfs, but early motor development slow.

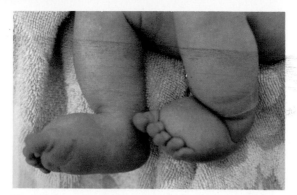

Fig. 103 Lymphoedema of feet in Turner's syndrome.

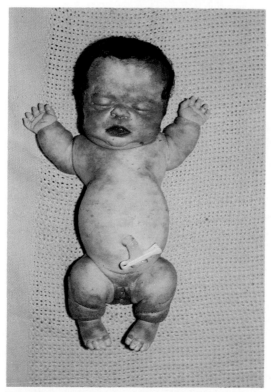

Fig. 104 Asphyxiating thoracic dystrophy.

Potter's syndrome

Synonym	Renal agenesis.
Incidence	1 in 3 000 live births.
Aetiology	The classical syndrome described by Potter was due to renal agenesis of unknown aetiology. Other renal defects (polycystic kidneys or chronic urinary tract obstruction) or chronic leakage of amniotic fluid, may also give rise to oligohydramnios and similar clinical manifestations.
Inheritance	Sporadic occurrence.
Clinical features	Low birth weight. Low set ears (Fig. 105). Compression abnormalities with flexion contractures of limbs. Hypoplastic lungs. Renal failure.
Course and prognosis	Renal insufficiency and progressive biochemical derangement occurs. Death is normally due to respiratory failure soon after birth.

Prune-belly syndrome

Incidence	Uncommon.
Inheritance	Sporadic occurrence.
Clinical features	Deficient abdominal wall musculature giving a rugose, prune-belly appearance (Fig. 106). Undescended testis. Multiple renal abnormalities.
Management	Surgical management of renal abnormalities if appropriate. Reconstitution of abdominal wall at a later stage.
Prognosis	Depends on the severity of renal abnormalities.

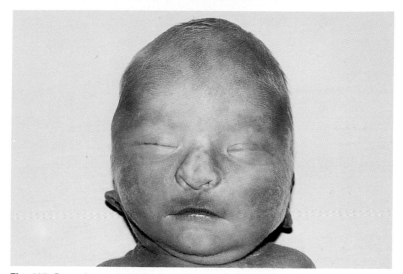

Fig. 105 Potter's syndrome.
(By courtesy of Dr G. Gau.)

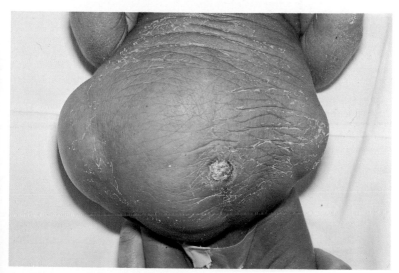

Fig. 106 Prune-belly syndrome with lax abdominal wall musculature.

Adrenogenital syndrome

Synonym
Congenital adrenal hyperplasia (CAH).

Incidence
1 in 5 000 for 21-hydroxylase deficiency. The other enzyme defects are much rarer.

Aetiology
This group of disorders is caused by absence of essential enzymes in the pathway of cortisol and aldosterone synthesis. As a result there is androgen excess. The commonest variety is due to 21-hydroxylase deficiency.

Inheritance
Autosomal recessive.

Clinical features
Affected females are virilised at birth and may be confused for males with hypospadias and cryptorchidism (Figs 107 & 108). Male infants may not be diagnosed until they develop an adrenal crisis in the second week of life, with vomiting and weight loss.

Investigation
A salt-losing adrenal crisis will be associated with hyponatraemia and hyperkalaemia. Grossly elevated serum 17-hydroxyprogesterone suggests the diagnosis of 21-hydroxylase deficiency. Elevated urinary pregnanetriol and 17-oxosteroids will confirm the diagnosis.

Management
Urgent intravenous saline will be required to treat a severe salt-losing crisis. The aim of long-term management is to suppress the hyperplastic adrenal glands and to provide physiological replacement of glucocorticoids and mineralocorticoids with hydrocortisone and fludrocortisone.
The masculinised female infant may require plastic surgery in early childhood.

Prognosis
Correct replacement therapy will ensure normal linear growth. Hydrocortisone and fludrocortisone replacement is required for life.

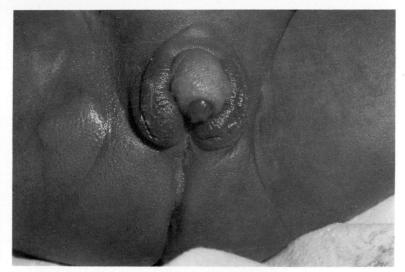

Fig. 107 Enlarged clitoris in adrenogenital syndrome.

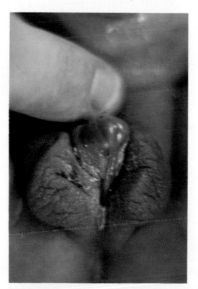

Fig. 108 Enlarged clitoris and rugose labia majora which could be confused with severe hypospadias.

Osteogenesis imperfecta

Synonym Brittle bone disease.

Incidence Uncommon.

Inheritance The severe congenital broad-boned type of osteogenesis imperfecta is usually autosomal recessive. Other less severe forms may be autosomal dominant.

Aetiology Unknown; there appears to be an abnormality of collagen formation.

Clinical features Poorly mineralised skull and long bones with multiple fractures and callus formation. In the severe form, they often have short, deformed limbs at birth due to intra-uterine fractures (Figs 109 & 110). Crepitus may be felt in bones with recent fractures. Blue sclerae are sometimes present, but may be difficult to diagnose in the neonatal period.

Prognosis There is wide variability in the natural history of the disorder, with stillbirth or early mortality among severely affected infants. Beyond infancy, the outlook for survival is good, but the child is often handicapped by orthopaedic deformity and deafness secondary to otosclerosis.

Management Careful nursing is mandatory. Orthopaedic treatment of fractures is the only form of treatment that can be offered, but optimal management will limit deformity.

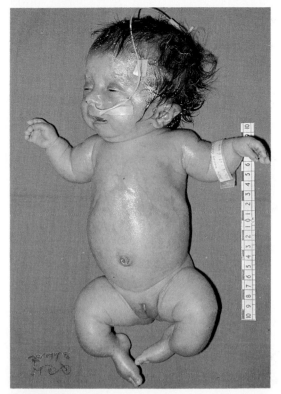

Fig. 109 Osteogenesis imperfecta.

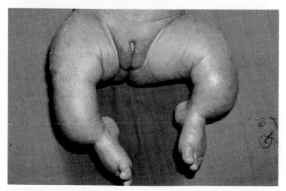

Fig. 110 Legs of a baby who had intra-uterine fractures from osteogenesis imperfecta.

Syndromes (7)

Congenital hypothyroidism

Synonym	Cretinism.
Incidence	1 in 6000 live births.
Aetiology	Defective thyroid gland development, occasionally secondary to maternal goitrogens or inborn errors of thyroxine synthesis.
Clinical features	Coarse facies and large protruding tongue (Figs 111 & 112). Hoarse cry. Poor weight gain. Umbilical hernia (Figs 112 & 113). Constipation. Prolonged jaundice. Hypothermia. Absence of spontaneous activity and crying. Feeding difficulties.
Associations	Rarely, a goitre may occur when hypothyroidism is secondary to maternal goitrogens or an inborn error of thyroxine synthesis.
Management	Thyroid hormone replacement for life.
Prognosis	Early diagnosis and treatment within 2 months of birth improves the outlook for normal mental development in the majority of cases. Routine screening of all infants within a few days of birth will enable early diagnosis and reduce morbidity.

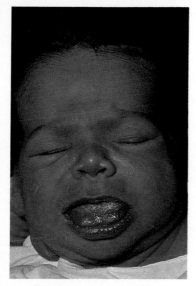

Fig. 111 Coarse facies and large protruding tongue of congenital hypothyroidism.

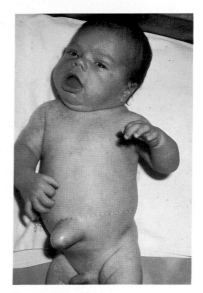

Fig. 112 Umbilical hernia and large tongue.

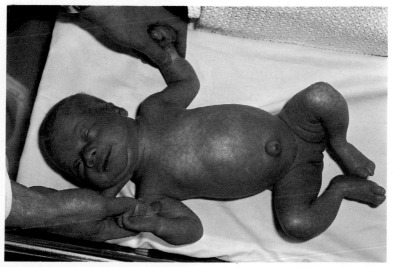

Fig. 113 Congenital hypothyroidism.

Pierre Robin syndrome

Synonym	Robin anomalad.
Incidence	Relatively common.
Inheritance	Usually sporadic occurrence.
Aetiology	Early developmental anomaly with mandibular hypoplasia, posterior location of the tongue and impaired closure of the posterior palate.
Clinical features	Severe micrognathia (Fig. 114). Wide posterior midline cleft palate (Fig. 115).
Complications	Acute respiratory obstruction because of a tendency for the tongue to fall back into the cleft palate; feeding difficulties.
Management	Expert nursing is required, often with the infant in the face-down posture to prevent respiratory obstruction. Surgical closure of the cleft palate should be performed after 3 months of age.
Course and prognosis	High mortality in early infancy due to acute respiratory obstruction. Micrognathia and glossoptosis improve during infancy.

Klippel-Feil syndrome

Incidence	About 1 in 40 000 live births; female predominance.
Inheritance	Sporadic occurrence of unknown aetiology.
Clinical features	There is a short immobile neck, secondary webbing of neck, low hair-line (Fig. 116) and fusion of cervical vertebrae. Hemivertebrae, rib defects, scoliosis and Sprengel's shoulder sometimes occur.
Associations	Deafness in approximately 30% of cases. The syndrome may occur as part of a more serious defect of neural tube development.

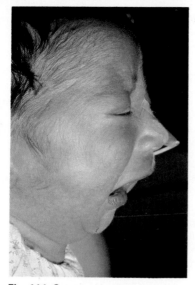

Fig. 114 Severe micrognathia of Pierre Robin syndrome.

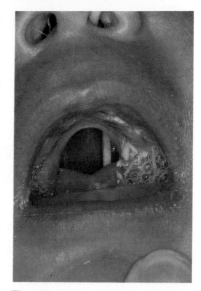

Fig. 115 Wide posterior midline cleft palate.

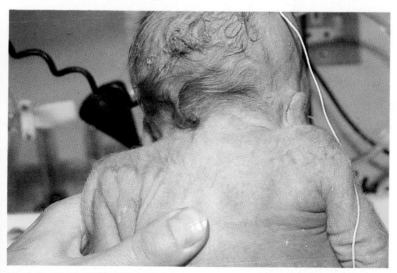

Fig. 116 Short neck and low hair line in Klippel—Feil syndrome.

6 | Syndromes (9)

Infant of diabetic mother

Incidence
Good control of maternal diabetes throughout pregnancy reduces the signs and symptoms in infants of diabetic mothers, except the increased risk of congenital abnormalities.

Clinical features
Large obese infants (Figs 117 & 118) who often develop respiratory distress syndrome. After birth, there is a risk of hypoglycaemia due to islet cell hyperplasia, and polycythaemia.

Management
Infants of diabetic mothers require careful observation in the first few hours after birth, with regular monitoring of blood sugar. Hypoglycaemia usually responds to frequent milk feeds or an intravenous infusion of dextrose.

Course and prognosis
The hypoglycaemia settles within a few days and provided it has been recognised and treated adequately, will not give rise to any sequelae.

Prevention
The frequency of congenital abnormalities (5%) is higher than the general population risk (3%). It is not yet known whether meticulous diabetic control before conception will reduce this high risk.

Beckwith's syndrome

Incidence
Rare.

Aetiology
Unknown.

Inheritance
Usually sporadic occurrence.

Clinical features
Large birth weight infants with glossoptosis (Fig. 119) and omphalocele. Hypoglycaemia due to pancreatic hyperplasia and polycythaemia often occur.

Prognosis
High mortality in the neonatal period.

NEONATOLOGY

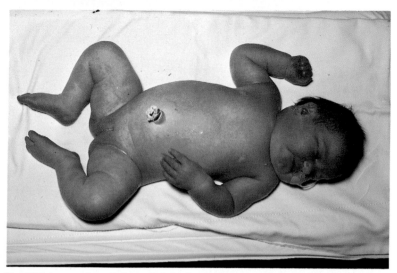

Fig. 117 Large obese infant of diabetic mother.

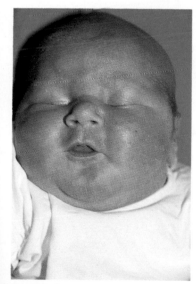

Fig. 118 Cherubic facies of infant of diabetic mother.

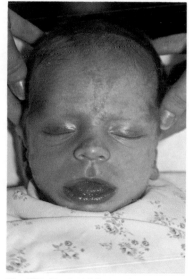

Fig. 119 Beckwith's syndrome with glossoptosis.

Hydrops fetalis

Incidence	Uncommon: less common since the prevention of rhesus disease with anti-D.
Aetiology	Haemolytic disease, particularly rhesus isoimmunisation. α-Thalassaemia. Intra-uterine viral infections, particularly cytomegalovirus. Congenital syphilis. Supraventricular tachycardia with congestive cardiac failure. Congenital nephrotic syndrome.
Clinical features	Pallor. Gross generalised oedema (Figs 120 & 121). Ascites. Pleural effusions. Congestive heart failure. Severe respiratory distress due to pulmonary oedema or pulmonary hypoplasia.
Management	Depends on the cause of hydrops. If hydrops is secondary to haemolytic disease, exchange transfusions and ventilatory support are the mainstay of treatment. In the presence of cardiac failure secondary to a tachyarrhythmia, treatment is directed towards correcting the arrhythmia with drugs or defibrillation, and supportive treatment of cardiac failure.
Prognosis	Depends on the underlying cause; prognosis is usually good if the infant survives the neonatal period.

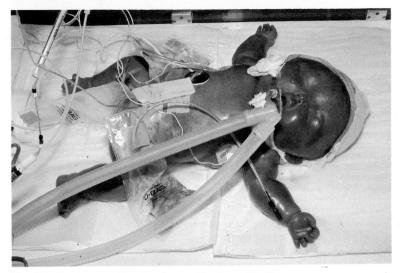

Fig. 120 Gross generalised oedema of hydrops fetalis.

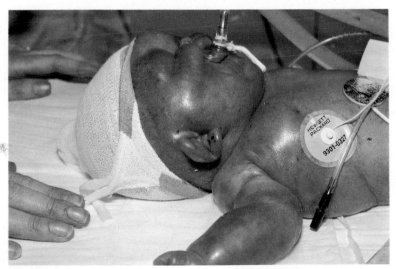

Fig. 121 Pallor and oedema in hydrops fetalis due to rhesus haemolytic disease.

Staphylococcal infection

Incidence

Serious staphylococcal infection is now uncommon, but minor superficial infections are not.

Aetiology

Bacterial infection caused by gram-positive cocci, *Staphylococcus aureus*.

Clinical features

Superficial staphylococcal infections result in small pustules anywhere on the skin (Figs 122 & 123). Umbilical sepsis (Fig. 124) is very common and if there is a frank discharge or peri-umbilical cellulitis, systemic antibiotics will be required. Paronychiae of the fingers and toes, although apparently minor infections, may cause more serious sepsis if not promptly treated. Occasionally toxic epidermal necrolysis (TEN, scalded skin syndrome or Ritter's disease) with extensive epidermal separation may develop (Fig. 125).

Complications

Septicaemia; meningitis; osteomyelitis.

Management

All superficial infections in young infants should be promptly treated with broad-spectrum systemic antibiotics after appropriate swabs and cultures.

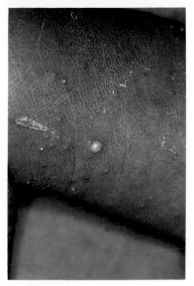

Fig. 122 Staphylococcal pustule.

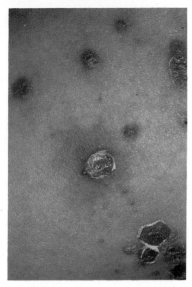

Fig. 123 Impetiginous staphylococcal lesions.

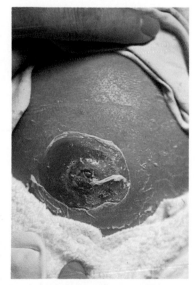

Fig. 124 Peri-umbilical cellulitis.

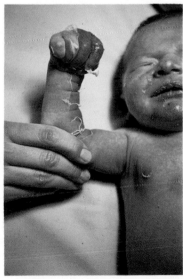

Fig. 125 Toxic epidermal necrolysis.

Ophthalmitis

Incidence

Minor sticky eye is extremely common.

Aetiology

Conjunctivitis may be due to a variety of organisms, the most serious being the sexually transmitted *Neiserria gonorrhoea* and *Chlamydia trachomatis*.

Clinical features

Manifestations vary from a mild sticky eye (Fig. 126), to severe conjunctival inflammation with pussy discharge and peri-orbital oedema. Gonococcal ophthalmitis causes severe signs within 48 h of birth (Fig. 127). Chlamydia infection (Fig. 128) often does not become apparent until the second week of life and may co-exist with gonorrhoea.

Diagnosis

Appropriate swabs should be taken, but treatment should be commenced immediately if gonorrhoea is suspected.

Management

Minor sticky eyes are usually non-infective and respond to saline eye washes. Gonococcal ophthalmitis should be treated with high-dose penicillin, given both topically and systemically. *Chlamydia trachomatis* infection will be eradicated with chlortetracycline eye ointment and systemic erythromycin. Most other minor infections will respond to neomycin or chloramphenicol eye drops or ointment. When gonorrhoea or chlamydia are diagnosed, both parents will require genital swabs and treatment.

Complications

Inadequate treatment of gonorrhoea ophthalmitis may lead to corneal scarring and blindness. In Third World countries, chlamydia frequently causes blindness from trachoma, but this is uncommon in developed countries. The reason for this different outcome from the same organism is unclear.

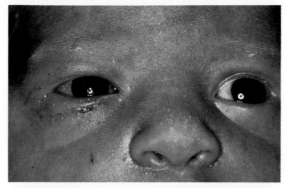

Fig. 126 Minor sticky eye with conjunctival inflammation.

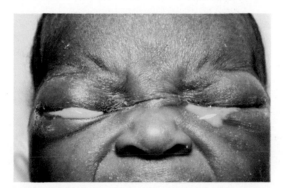

Fig. 127 Frank pus discharge in gonococcal ophthalmitis.

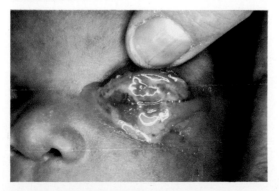

Fig. 128 Chlamydia ophthalmitis.

Thrush

Synonyms	Monilia, candida.
Incidence	Superficial infection of the mouth or perineum is extremely common, particularly after antibiotic therapy.
Aetiology	Fungal infection caused by *Candida albicans*.
Clinical features	Oral or perineal thrush is usually a trivial, but distressing superficial infection. In the mouth, it appears as white plaques which cannot be wiped off without causing bleeding (Fig. 129). Sometimes on visual inspection, it may be difficult to distinguish from milk immediately after a feed, but milk can always be easily wiped off. Perineal thrush gives a bright red confluent rash in the napkin area or around the anus. Typically there are discrete ulcerated satellite lesions lying peripheral to the confluent rash (Fig. 130).
Management	Swabs or scrapings should be taken to confirm the diagnosis, although it is usually clinically obvious. Superficial thrush responds rapidly to topical nystatin or miconazole. Systemic candidiasis, though uncommon, may occur in ill preterm infants and responds poorly to antifungal agents.

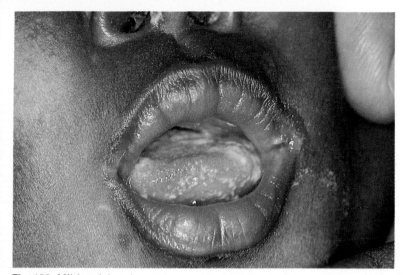

Fig. 129 Mild oral thrush.

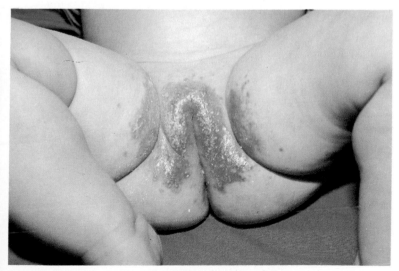

Fig. 130 Perineal monilia with satellite lesions.

Congenital rubella

Synonym	Rubella embryopathy.
Incidence	Depends on the state of immunity of the child-bearing population and the occurrence of rubella epidemics in the community.
Aetiology	Rubella virus infection; severe abnormalities occur with infection before 12 weeks' gestation.
Clinical features	Growth retardation with mental deficiency and microcephaly, deafness, cataracts, microphthalmia and congenital heart disease occur in severely affected infants (Fig. 131). Hepatosplenomegaly, anaemia, thrombocytopenic purpura (Fig. 132) and osteolytic lesions in long bones may be present.
Prevention	Mass rubella immunisation of susceptible individuals is recommended to reduce the frequency of rubella embryopathy.

Neonatal herpes infection

Incidence	Uncommon.
Aetiology	Herpes hominus, usually type II virus, which is acquired by the infant during delivery through a genital tract with active herpes infection.
Clinical features	A generalised vesicular eruption (Fig. 133) occurs and if encephalitis occurs, mortality is very high.
Prognosis	There is a high risk of neurological abnormality and mental retardation amongst survivors.
Treatment	Systemic antiviral agents (acyclovir) may be helpful if commenced early in the disease.
Prevention	Elective Caesarean section should be considered if active maternal genital herpes has been present in late pregnancy.

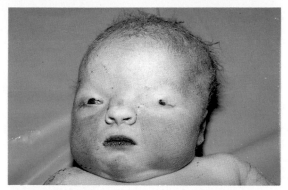

Fig. 131 Microphthalmia.

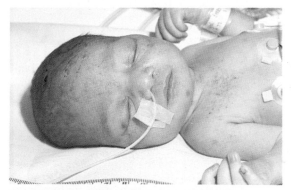

Fig. 132 Thrombocytopenic purpura in rubella embryopathy.

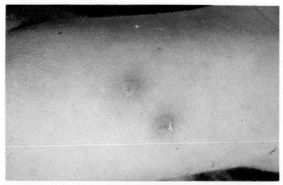

Fig. 133 Typical herpetic lesions.

Cytomegalovirus (CMV) and toxoplasmosis

Incidence

In the UK, 1% of newborn infants excrete CMV in urine; the majority are asymptomatic. Toxoplasmosis is less common.

Transmission

Infected adults usually suffer only a mild flu-like illness. Toxoplasmosis is acquired from eating infected raw meat or from cat faeces.

Clinical features

Infected infants (Fig. 134) often have hepatosplenomegaly, lymphadenopathy, thrombocytopenic purpura, jaundice, growth retardation, intracranial calcification and chorioretinitis. Hydrocephalus is common in toxoplasmosis; microcephaly occurs more often with CMV infection. Deafness, mental retardation and epilepsy may occur later.

Management

There is no effective treatment. Pyrimethamine and sulphadiazine may be used in congenital toxoplasmosis if active eye lesions are present.

Prognosis

Variable; the majority of infants with CMV infection develop no sequelae; 5% develop deafness; 1% show more serious neurological manifestations.

Congenital chicken pox

Incidence

Rare; fetus will be immune if mother has had chicken pox.

Clinical features

Infant may have scars if infected in utero (Fig. 135). Neonatal chicken pox is particularly severe, and hyperimmune zoster globulin should be administered to the infant at birth if maternal chicken pox or a close contact is likely.

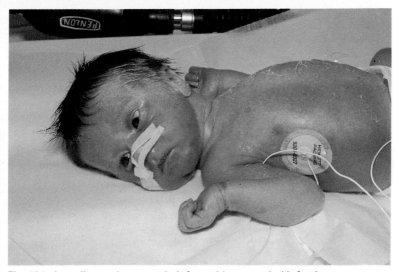

Fig. 134 Jaundice and purpura in infant with congenital infection.

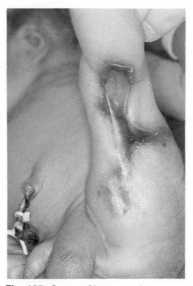

Fig. 135 Scars of intra-uterine chicken pox.

Umbilical hernia

Incidence

Common: 20% of all newborn infants and 60% negroid infants. Higher incidence in preterm.

Clinical features

Central defect in the abdominal wall at the insertion of the umbilicus, with herniation of bowel into the redundant umbilical skin (Fig. 136). On crying, straining or coughing, the skin covering the bowel-filled hernia often becomes tense, shiny and bluish. It is not painful, but becomes more pronounced with crying. Umbilical herniae always reduce easily when the infant is lying quietly or when asleep.

Significance

Cosmetic deformity only. Strangulation is extremely rare in central umbilical herniae, but may occur in para-umbilical herniae (defect in the linea alba separate from, but adjacent to the umbilicus).

Management

Most close spontaneously within the first few years of life. Strapping does not hasten spontaneous resolution. Cosmetic surgery is occasionally required.

Umbilical granuloma

Incidence

Common.

Clinical features

A soft, spongy, often pedunculated pink umbilical mass (Fig. 137), which is sometimes accompanied by a sero-sanguinous discharge.

Differential diagnosis

Careful inspection should exclude a persistent urachus or omphalo-mesenteric remnant.

Management

Application of silver nitrate to the granuloma or the pedunculated base until resolution occurs. Surgical excision is occasionally required.

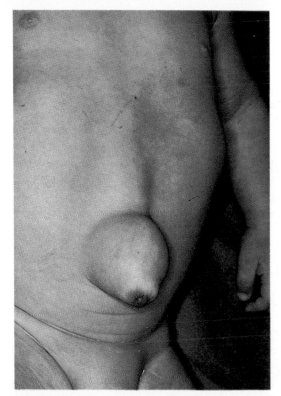

Fig. 136 Umbilical hernia and divarication of the recti.

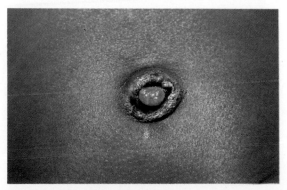

Fig. 137 Umbilical granuloma.

8 | Surgical Problems (2)

Inguinal hernia

Incidence

Indirect inguinal hernia is the commonest condition requiring surgery during infancy—1 in 50 live male births, with the greatest incidence in the first 3 months in life.

Aetiology

Persistent patency of the processus vaginalis, accompanied by herniation of small bowel.

Clinical features

Intermittent swelling in the inguinal region or scrotum, often noticed after crying or straining (Fig. 138). Herniae are usually easily reducible, but when they become irreducible there is a high risk of strangulation.

Management

Surgical repair should be done as soon as practicable after the diagnosis of an uncomplicated hernia, because the risk of strangulation is high in young infants. Strangulation with a tense, tender, irreducible swelling sometimes accompanied by vomiting, abdominal distension and signs of gut obstruction, is an indication for immediate surgery.

Hydrocele

Incidence

Common.

Aetiology

Patency of the processus vaginalis.

Clinical features

An hydrocele is a painless, fluid-filled cyst anterior to the testis. The testis can usually be easily palpated within the scrotum. The hydrocele is brightly translucent (Fig. 139) and cannot be emptied by pressure although it may vary in size. The swelling can be diffentiated from a hernia because it does not extend up to the inguinal ring.

Management

The majority of hydroceles in infancy resolve spontaneously within the first year of life.

NEONATOLOGY

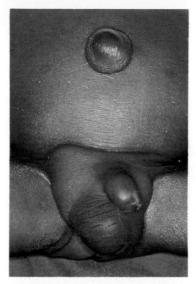

Fig. 138 Bilateral inguinal hernia and umbilical hernia.

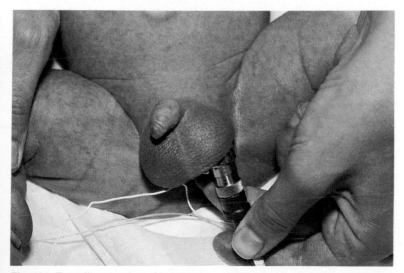

Fig. 139 Transillumination of hydrocele.

Hypospadias

Incidence

Glandular hypospadias is common (1 in 350 male infants).

Clinical features

The urethral orifice is situated on the ventral aspect of the penis at a site proximal to the normal opening (Fig. 140), with severity varying from a glandular orifice to a scrotal or perineal site. Hypospadias is usually accompanied by a redundant dorsal hooded prepuce (due to failure of fusion of the ventral foreskin) and is sometimes associated with ventral curvature called chordee (Fig. 141).

Management

Mild glandular hypospadias without chordee is usually insignifiant and surgery is not required unless there is meatal stenosis. Surgical repair is indicated if the orifice is situated proximal to the glans or if chordee is present: this can only be judged when the baby has an erection. Circumcision should be delayed until corrective surgery is performed, as the prepuce may be required for urethroplasty.

Ectopia vesicae

Incidence

Very rare; more common in males.

Clinical features

Wide separation of the pubic symphysis with ventral herniation of the bladder, exposure of the bladder mucosa and a deficiency of the pelvic floor leading to rectal prolapse (Fig. 142). Often accompanied by epispadias, undescended testis and an inguinal hernia. In the female, the clitoris is frequently septate or duplicated. Abnormalities of the kidneys are common.

Management

Surgical reconstruction is difficult. Continence is rarely achieved.

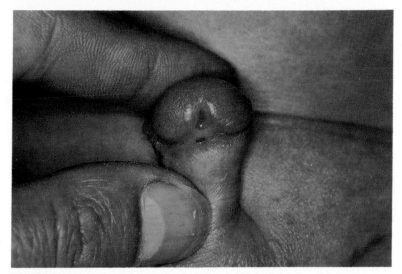

Fig. 140 Hypospadias with urethral orifice on shaft of penis.

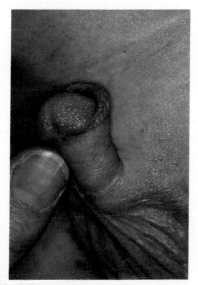

Fig. 141 Hypospadias with dorsal hooded prepuce.

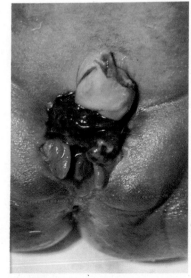

Fig. 142 Ectopia vesicae.

Necrotising enterocolitis (NEC)

Incidence

Variable; more common in preterm infants. Has been found to be associated with birth asphyxia, umbilical catheterisation, early feeding and artificial milk formulae. Clusters of cases may occur.

Aetiology

Unknown; probably related to gut ischaemia and secondary infection with invasion by gut flora.

Pathology

Histological evidence of impaired gut perfusion, bowel ischaemia and necrosis, usually affecting the terminal ileum, caecum and proximal transverse colon.

Clinical features

Abdominal distension, vomiting and the passage of bloody stools. NEC is sometimes accompanied by peritonitis, oedema of the anterior abdominal wall, dilated abdominal veins or a palpable mass (Fig. 143).

Invasion by gas-forming organisms or diffusion of intraluminal gas into the bowel wall gives rise to the pathognomonic sign of pneumatosis intestinalis (intramural bubbles of gas) on plain abdominal X-ray (Figs 144 & 145).

Management

Oral feeds should be discontinued and parenteral nutrition may be required. Antibiotics, including those for anaerobes, are usually given but specific pathogens are rarely isolated. Analgesia and naso-gastric suction may be indicated.

Perforation is the only indication for laparotomy in the acute stages of NEC when mortality is high with surgery.

Course and prognosis

With conservative management, the mortality has improved, but gut obstruction secondary to adhesions or stricture may require surgical intervention at a later state in approximately 25% of survivors.

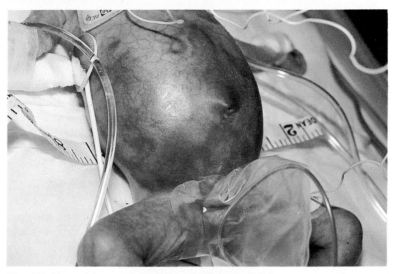

Fig. 143 Necrotising enterocolitis with distended abdomen.

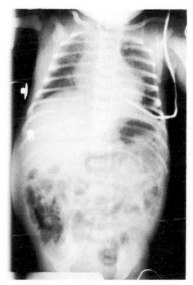

Fig. 144 X-ray showing intramural gas.

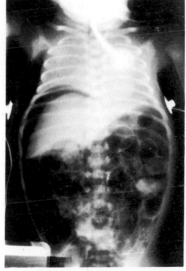

Fig. 145 X-ray showing gas in the peritoneal cavity from perforation.

Exomphalos

Synonym	Omphalocele.
Incidence	Uncommon.
Aetiology	Unknown.
Pathology	Failure of rotation and re-entry of gut into abdominal cavity during fetal development.
Clinical features	Congenital herniation of abdominal viscera through midline abdominal wall defect with umbilical cord at apex, and sometimes with a covering of peritoneum (Figs 146 & 147). Exomphalos can be differentiated from gastroschisis where there is no sac, and the umbilical cord is inserted at the edge of the defect.
Associations	Other congenital abnormalities are common, particularly cardiac or bowel defects.
Management	Surgical closure as soon as possible. The bowel should first be carefully inspected for stenosis or atresia which often accompany exomphalos. With large defects, definitive repair is often delayed until the peritoneal cavity is able to accommodate the contents. The sac and contents are usually enclosed in an artificial membrane, which is gradually reduced in size over a period of some weeks, as the contents are slowly replaced into the abdominal cavity.

NEONATOLOGY

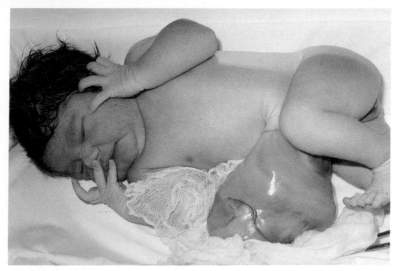

Fig. 146 Exomphalos with peritoneal covering.

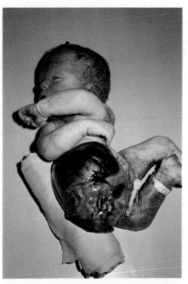

Fig. 147 Massive exomphalos with herniation of entire abdominal contents.

Imperforate anus

Synonyms Anal atresia, covered anus, rectal atresia.

Clinical features Imperforate anus (Figs 148 & 149) is usually diagnosed during routine examination immediately after birth, but occasionally presents later as intestinal obstruction or delayed passage of meconium.

Associations Other congenital abnormalities are found in approximately 60% of cases. Recto-genito-urinary fistulae are common, particularly in high rectal atresia. Urinary tract infections are common, particularly when there is a fistula.

Management In the simplest cases, the covering of the anus can be incised. In the more usual cases, colostomy is performed in the neonatal period. A thorough search should be made for fistulae, particularly in females. Rectoplasty and a pull-through procedure are done later, at 6–12 months of age. Continence is achieved in approximately 70% of cases after final surgery.

Vaginal defects

Incidence Uncommon.

Clinical features Imperforate hymen is a rare condition which may present in the neonatal period with an accumulation of mucus beneath the imperforate membrane (mucocolpos) which bulges out between the labia minora. Paravaginal cysts (Fig. 150) may be confused with an imperforate hymen, but it is possible to pass a probe into the vagina alongside the cyst.

Management Imperforate hymen requires surgical drainage and excision of the membrane. Paravaginal cysts usually rupture spontaneously.

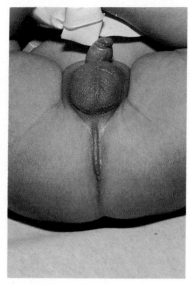

Fig. 148 Imperforate anus.

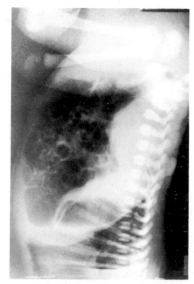

Fig. 149 X-ray showing imperforate anus with high rectal atresia.

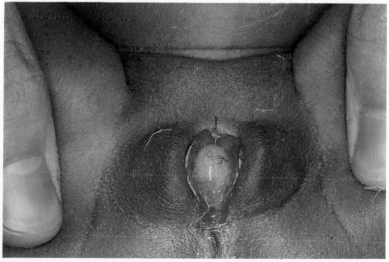

Fig. 150 Paravaginal cyst.

Diaphragmatic hernia

Incidence 1 in 1 500 live births.

Aetiology Failure of fusion or muscularisation of the anterior and posterior leaves of the diaphragm; most commonly due to persistence of the pleuro-peritoneal canal, usually on the left side and resulting in a postero-lateral hernia through the foramen of Bochdalek.

Clinical features Most diaphragmatic herniae are large and produce cardio-respiratory symptoms soon after birth. The signs and symptoms depend on the size of the hernia and include respiratory distress, cyanosis, dextrocardia and scaphoid abdomen with reduced or absent abdominal contents (Fig. 151).

Associations Pulmonary hypoplasia; gut anomalies.

Management Confirm the diagnosis with CXR (Fig. 152). Urgent surgical repair of the diaphragmatic defect and replacement of the abdominal contents will be necessary. Pre-operative decompression of the gut with a large naso-gastric tube and mechanical ventilation may be required.

Prognosis Mortality is high (approximately 40%) even after successful surgery. Survival depends on the severity of pulmonary hypoplasia.

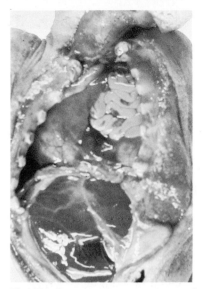

Fig. 151 Post-mortem appearance of diaphragmatic hernia (by courtesy of Dr S. Gould).

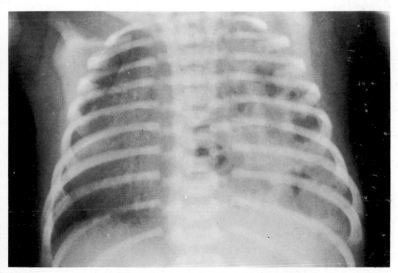

Fig. 152 X-ray appearance of typical left-sided diaphragmatic hernia.

Preterm

Definition

Immature, less than 37 weeks' gestation and birth weight usually less than 2 500 g. The very premature require intensive care (Fig. 153).

Incidence

In the UK, approx. 6–7% of live births are of low birth weight (less than 2 500 g). About two-thirds of these are preterm infants.

Aetiology

Often unknown; sometimes the infant has to be delivered early because of maternal complications of pregnancy such as pre-eclampsia or placenta praevia. Premature labour is often associated with cervical incompetence, multiple pregnancy, premature rupture of the membranes or amnionitis.

Clinical features

It is possible to make an estimate of gestational age from a combination of external physical and neurological signs. The preterm infant has poor muscle tone and tends to lie in a frog-like position. He has a relatively large head and prominent abdomen. Because the skull bones are soft and poorly mineralised, the head of the preterm infant often becomes narrow and elongated (Fig. 154), particularly if he is nursed with his head to one side. This deformity of the shape of the skull resolves spontaneously in later infancy and is of no significance.

Skin creases are poorly developed, particularly on the soles of the feet (Fig. 155). Lanugo hair is often profuse in babies of 30–36 weeks' gestation, but is less common in very preterm or more mature infants. It is usually most pronounced over the back and shoulders, but may occur all over the body (Fig. 156). Ear cartilage is soft and

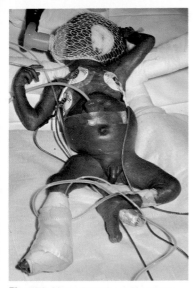

Fig. 153 Very preterm infant with some equipment of modern intensive care.

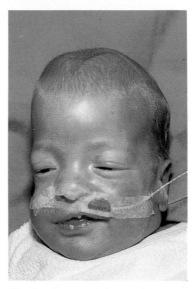

Fig. 154 Preterm infant with narrow, elongated head.

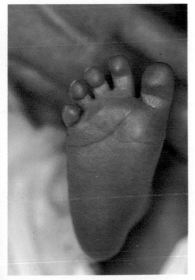

Fig. 155 Poorly developed skin creases on feet.

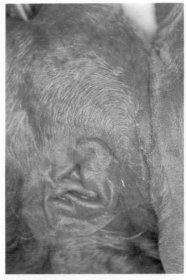

Fig. 156 Profuse lanugo and primitive ear development.

Preterm
(contd)

Clinical features (contd)

deficient and the pinna is poorly developed (Fig. 156), with little elastic recoil. The skin is often bright red, shiny and transparent with subcutaneous blood vessels readily visible (Fig. 157). The skin of the preterm infant is easily damaged by even minor trauma such as adhesive tape or transcutaneous electrodes.

The nipple does not appear until 28 weeks' gestation and breast tissue does not develop until after 34 weeks' gestation. The genitalia show major changes with advancing gestation. In female infants, the clitoris is relatively large with gaping of the vulva due to prominent labia majora (Fig. 158). In male infants, the scrotum is under-developed, and the testes may be undescended (Fig. 159).

Complications and associations

Respiratory distress syndrome (hyaline membrane disease).
Intraventricular haemorrhage.
Poor temperature control.
Increased susceptibility to infection.
Severe and prolonged physiological jaundice.
Feeding difficulties and inability to suck.
Fluid and electrolyte imbalance.

Course and prognosis

Mortality is still high in very preterm infants. Survival is unlikely under 24 weeks' gestation, but 60% infants survive at 28 weeks and 95% at 30 weeks and over. With optimal care, more than 90% preterm infants who survive the neonatal period have no serious neurological handicap.

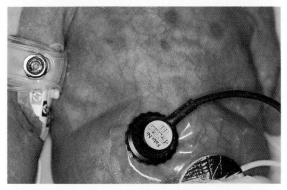

Fig. 157 Transparent, easily traumatised skin with prominent veins.

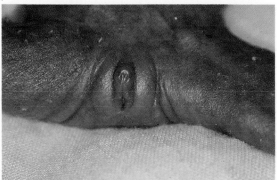

Fig. 158 Immature female genitalia with prominent labia minora and enlarged clitoris.

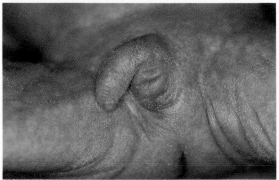

Fig. 159 Immature male genitalia with under-developed scrotum and undescended testes.

Small for gestational age (SGA)

Synonym	Small for dates (SFD); intra-uterine growth retardation (IUGR).
Definition	Birth weight less than 10th centile for gestational age.
Incidence	2 in 100 live births are both SGA, and less than 2 500 g.
Aetiology	May be associated with placental insufficiency, maternal pre-eclampsia, hypertension, smoking or intra-uterine infection such as rubella.
Clinical features	The commonest SGA infants are usually long and thin, with dry peeling skin (Fig. 160) and long nails. Their physical appearance and behaviour are appropriate for gestational age, not birth weight. Some SGA are uniformly small; they are at risk of perinatal asphyxia and often have meconium staining of the skin (Fig. 161), nails and umbilical cord. Unless they are ill, SGA infants feed very well and require increased caloric intake. Their physiological weight loss is usually insignificant and they gain weight rapidly with adequate postnatal nutrition. They are at risk of hypoglycaemia in the first few days after birth because of poor glycogen stores. Hypothermia may also occur because of lack of subcutaneous fat.
Course and prognosis	In the absence of intra-uterine infection or neonatal hypoglycaemia, SGA infants are usually of normal intelligence and development. Infants of low birth weight but appropriate head circumference and length for gestation usually achieve normal centiles for all aspects of growth later. If the head circumference, weight and length are all low at birth indicating long-standing intra-uterine growth retardation, postnatal growth may always remain below the normal centiles.

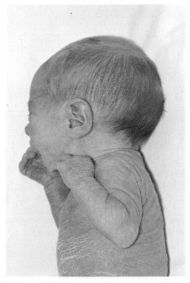

Fig. 160 Dry peeling skin of SGA infant.

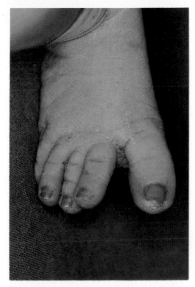

Fig. 161 Meconium staining of skin and nails.

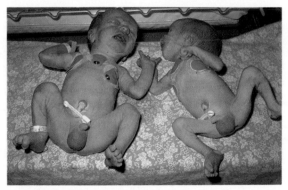

Fig. 162 SGA and normal twins.

Hyaline membrane disease

Synonyms	HMD; respiratory distress syndrome, RDS.
Incidence	Commonest neonatal respiratory disease. Gestational age is the main determinant of HMD; at least 50% of infants less than 32 weeks' gestation develop the disease. 70% of infants with a lecithin/sphingomyelin (L : S) ratio less than 1.5 : 1 develop HMD; it is extremely rare if the L : S ratio is greater than 2 : 1.
Aetiology	Due to surfactant deficiency in the infant's lungs. HMD is more likely to develop in infants who suffer perinatal asphyxia and infants of diabetic mothers.
Clinical features	HMD presents with respiratory distress within 4 h of birth. The infant usually has tachypnoea greater than 60/min, an expiratory grunt, cyanosis, and sternal, intercostal and subcostal recession (Fig. 163). After 4 h of age, HMD can usually be clearly distinguished from transient tachypnoea due to delayed lung liquid resorption, by a characteristic radiological appearance. CXR shows a diffuse reticulo-granular pattern due to atelectasis, and an air-bronchogram due to the air-filled major airways standing out as radiolucent areas (Fig. 164). In more serious HMD, the heart border may become obscured.
Course and prognosis	HMD gradually gets worse over the first 24–36 h, as the infant tires, and if there are no complications, steadily improves from 48 h onwards as surfactant is produced. The majority of infants with uncomplicated HMD recover by 7–10 days of age.

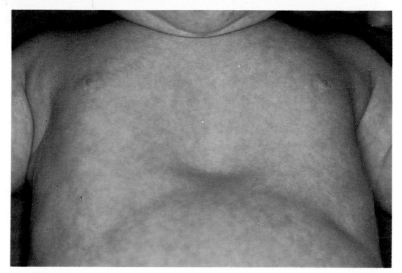

Fig. 163 Subcostal recession.

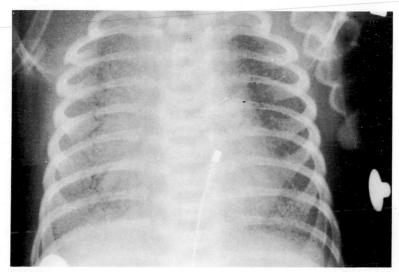

Fig. 164 X-ray appearance of hyaline membrane disease.

Hyaline membrane disease (contd)

Complications

Pneumothorax (Fig. 165) develops in up to 20% of infants with HMD, particularly if ventilation is required. In a small percentage of infants, pulmonary interstitial emphysema (PIE) (Fig. 166), pneumomediastinum (Fig. 167), pneumopericardium or bronchopulmonary dysplasia (BPD) may develop. Intraventricular haemorrhage (IVH) is the major cause of death in preterm infants with HMD. The haemorrhage arises from the capillaries of the extremely vascular germinal layer of the floor of the lateral ventricle. Of infants less than 1 500 g, 40% suffer from IVH, which can be detected on ultrasound examination of the brain. Germinal layer haemorrhage or small IVH is of no serious significance. Haemorrhage which distends the ventricles, extends into brain substance or causes post-haemorrhagic hydrocephalus may be fatal or cause long-term neurological sequelae.

Management

The aim is to keep the infant alive and in good condition until natural surfactant synthesis occurs. Hypoxia, acidosis and hypothermia will inhibit surfactant production. Oxygen and artificial ventilation are often necessary in order to maintain arterial PO_2 within the range 8–12 kPa (60–90 mmHg). Continuous monitoring of PaO_2 and frequent estimates of acid–base status are particularly important in the first few days when IVH often occurs.

Outcome

Survival and long-term prognosis depend on gestation and the occurrence of complications. With improvement in ventilatory techniques in the past decade, IVH is now the main determinant of survival and neurological handicap.
With optimal care, less than 10% of preterm infants suffer major handicap.

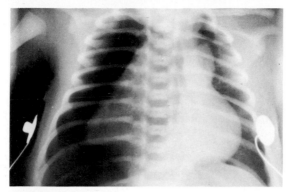

Fig. 165 Pneumothorax.

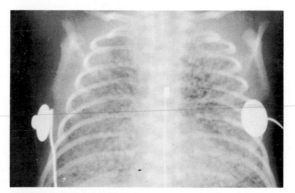

Fig. 166 Pulmonary interstitial emphysema.

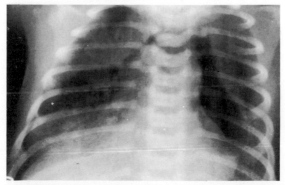

Fig. 167 Pneumomediastinum.

Nutrition

Breast feeding

The major advantage of breast milk over all formulae is its anti-infective properties. Fresh breast milk from the infant's own mother should be used whenever possible; pasteurisation probably kills the white cells, and most anti-infective factors are destroyed by boiling. Breast feeding (Fig. 168), or the use of expressed breast milk (EBM), is also psychologically important to the maternal–infant relationship. There are, however, physiological limitations on nutrition in low birth weight infants. Particular difficulties may occur with low gastric volume tolerance, poor fat absorption, high energy requirement, fluid and electrolyte imbalance in preterm infants.

Other feeding techniques

Many infants are unable to suck because of immaturity or respiratory distress. They can be fed through an indwelling naso-gastric tube, by intermittent gavage feeding (Fig. 170), or a continuous infusion of milk may be delivered via a syringe pump. Continuous transpyloric feeding (Fig. 169) may be useful if apnoea or vomiting occurs. Parenteral nutrition may be required in extremely small, immature or very sick infants whose gut may not tolerate milk feeds; it is best administered via a centrally placed silastic catheter introduced through a peripheral vein. Low birth weight infants usually require high protein and water intake for normal weight gain. Additional supplements of sodium, iron, vitamins, calcium, phosphate and folic acid are often necessary.

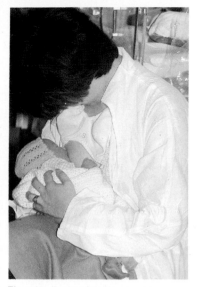

Fig. 168 Breast feeding preterm infant.

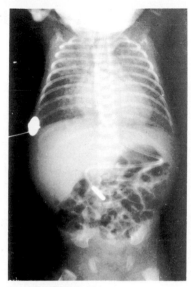

Fig. 169 Transpyloric tube for continuous milk infusion.

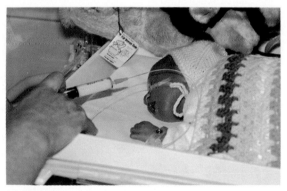

Fig. 170 Naso-gastric feeding.

The family

Parental anxiety

Guilt and a sense of failure often accompany the birth of a low birth weight infant. The appearance, behaviour and illness of a preterm infant may be difficult for the parents to accept and understand. Discussion and explanation of the infant's condition and management, including the awesome equipment of the modern neonatal unit, will help to alleviate some of the uncertainty faced by the family—even though an accurate prediction of outcome cannot be made in the early stages.

Avoidance of separation

Unnecessary admission of well, low birth weight infants to a specialised neonatal unit should be avoided whenever possible, as such admission always results in separation for some members of the family. Open visiting for all family members, including siblings (Figs 171 & 172) should be encouraged and some contribution towards active participation in the infant's care is usually possible and is always satisfying. This may include nursing, cuddling, nappy changing, bathing (Fig. 173) and feeding all but the most ill preterm infant.

Even in the event of the death of the baby, parents are often best supported by allowing them to participate in the final decisions and moments of the infant's life.

Later problems

The high incidence of feeding and managment problems is partly attributable to the immaturity of the infant and the fact that low birth weight infants are most often born to young mothers living in poor social conditions. With understanding and good support, many problems and parental anxieties can be overcome.

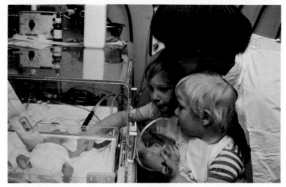

Fig. 171 Siblings visiting neonatal nursery.

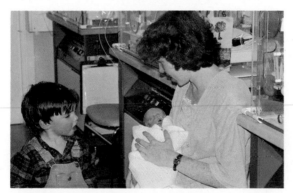

Fig. 172 Showing the baby to her brother.

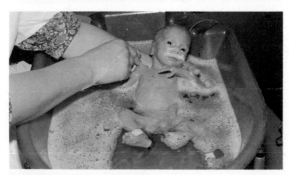

Fig 173 Bath-time.

116605 (S)